ADVANCE PRAISE FOR
GOT HEALTH-STYLE?

Being a health professional, [I know that] an active and clean-eating lifestyle is crucial to maintaining a healthy and injury-free body. Got Health-Style? is a perfect six-week guide to get anybody started on a path of positive and long-term well-being. Dr. Tichi provides you with powerful courage, motivation, . . . and an interactive journal to get you to your goals.

KRISTIN MAYNES PT, DPT
PHYSICAL THERAPIST

I am so impressed by Mary Tichi's work! She is truly a champion of life in so many ways. This is an amazing, well-put-together, inspirational health workbook which I strongly believe will change the life of so many individuals who struggle with creating a healthy lifestyle and healthy body. I cannot wait to share her work with all my patients.

DR. KATHY TOOSIE MD, FACS
BREAST CANCER SPECIALIST

[Got Health-Style? is a] very useful guide that can be advantageous to all people regardless of their levels of physical capabilities. A much-needed motivational aid that fills a void in the fitness and healthy lifestyles industry. A very personal piece that is relatable to a wide range of personalities.

PHIL SHUTTLEWORTH
FITNESS TRAINER AND HEAD COACH OF PLAYER DEVELOPMENT

Mary's book is, without a doubt, filling a huge need in the fitness industry. Weight loss and health are about so much more than eating right and hitting the gym, and Mary understands this. [Got Health-Style?] addresses the mental and emotional needs of [its] readers while still breaking down the basics of weight loss. I believe this book has the power to help people overcome a vast array of obstacles during their weight loss journey, and I recommend it to my personal training clients.

MEGAN LOONEY
NASM-CERTIFIED PERSONAL TRAINER AND FITNESS NUTRITION SPECIALIST

In the Got Health-Style? guide/workbook, Mary Tichi guides the reader in a physical and mental journey to health and fitness through self-inquiry by instruction and by example. Her authentic and compelling personal journal entries will truly encourage and inspire readers on their own path to resilience and well-being.

DR. RHONDA HONEYCUTT MS, PHD

As an executive coach I request that my clients declare a goal and design a passive accountability to accomplish that goal. Mary's book contains all the support and guidance—along with in-depth accountability—that you might need to accomplish your health and fitness goals, as well as to have fun on your journey. Her head, heart, and soul have been put into this guide, which provides additional inspiration along the way.

DAVE BROWN
NEXT LEVEL EXECUTIVE COACH

The battle of the bulge has been a long-time predicament for many people through the years. It is true—losing weight is not easy. Many weight-loss diets on the market claim their diet strategies are better than any other. However, your mindset is the most important factor for you to achieve your health and fitness goals! I know that this book will motivate and push you in order to reach your goals. In this guide you will discover . . . why you have to lose weight, get informed with weight-loss tips, and learn how to change your habits to achieve your goal that will help you keep the bulge off. [Readers will learn] to keep moving and [develop] the will power to get healthy and stay healthy. Mary is living proof that having your health and fitness goals is definitely worth a shot. Got Health-Style? will only make you healthier, fitter, and more motivated!

DR. SAMAN BAKHTIAR
PRESIDENT AND CO-FOUNDER OF THE CAMP TRANSFORMATION CENTER

GOT HEALTH-STYLE?

GOT HEALTH-STYLE?

A SIX-WEEK MOTIVATIONAL GUIDE FOR YOUR HEALTH AND FITNESS GOALS

YOU ARE NOT ALONE!

A 42-DAY JOURNEY IS SHARED WITH YOU ALONG THE WAY

MARY A. TICHI, PHD, MBA

MCP Books, Maitland, FL

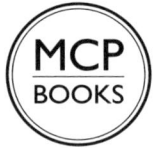

MCP Books
2301 Lucien Way #415
Maitland, FL 32751
407.339.4217
www.MCPBooks.com

ISBN-13: 978-1-63505-159-9
LCCN: 2016914777

Distributed by Itasca Books

Printed in the United States of America

CONTENTS

Written for all those who struggle with a healthy lifestyle
(Health-Style) path. You are not alone.

Dedicated to Dr. P. Humber, MD, my cancer surgeon, who inspired this project.
I hope to contribute, motivate, and make a difference, as you did for me.
Thank You. Rest in peace.

ACKNOWLEDGMENTS

I am eternally grateful to the fitness gym, The Camp Transformation Center, and to the owners, staff, trainers, numerous gym buddies, friends, and the whole "Awesome Fit Family" I met there. Your guidance and support in my own health and fitness journey encouraged my inner roar!

Special thanks to my husband, Steve, and my son, Dmitri. Your tender love and care carried me through the thick of it. You are the best team and support crew a wife and mama could ever wish for.

"Man sacrifices his health in order to make money. Then he sacrifices money to recuperate his health. And then he is so anxious about the future that he does not enjoy the present; the result being that he does not live in the present or the future; he lives as if he is never going to die, and then dies having never lived."

- James Lanchard

"It's your road . . . and yours alone . . . Others may walk it with you, but no one can walk it for you. No matter what path you choose, really walk it."

- Gautama Buddha

"In order to succeed, we must first believe that we can."

- Nikos Kazantzakis

I choose **MY PATH.**

I choose **TO BE AWARE OF THE PRESENT.**

I choose **TO LIVE NOW.**

I choose **MY HEALTH-STYLE.**

I am **STRONG.**

I am **COMMITTED.**

I am **DEDICATED.**

I will **PERSEVERE.**

I will **BE CHALLENGED.**

I will **SUCCEED.**

I can **DO THIS!**

INTRODUCTION

"A journey of a thousand miles begins with a single step"
– Lao Tzu

"No one stands at the beginning of a race and then finds himself at the end having never taken a step forward. And if that were to happen—the sweat and struggle avoided—what stories would he have to tell? The goal includes the journey; it's all part of the dream."
– Richelle E. Goodrich

CONGRATULATIONS! You are currently at an important and exciting turning point, about to build new habits and change your lifestyle for the better. Whether you have decided on a specific fitness goal, nutrition goal, weight loss goal, weight gain goal, endurance goal, strength goal, or *whatever* goal, it is a decision for change and action. A healthy lifestyle, or "health-style" (as I call it), can be yours for the taking.

Building new habits is a long-term venture, which takes repetition, time, dedication, and practice to achieve. A study published in *The European Journal of Social Psychology*[1] showed that, on average, it takes a little over two months for a behavior to become adopted and automatic for the long-term. This means that you need to have both short-term *and* long-term intentions in place in order to adopt new, lifelong, healthy habits.

By connecting with your inner strengths and specific motivational drivers, you can develop and implement your own strategies for changing your health-style for the better. This guide you hold in your hands is

---

1   Phillippa Lally, et al, "How are habits formed: Modeling habit formation in the real world," *European Journal of Social Psychology* 40, no. 6 (2010): 998-1009.

specifically designed to help you uncover the drivers which will ultimately lead to your long-term success. Throughout this journey you will be asked questions such as:

- **What underlying needs do you have?**
- **What are your strengths—and how can you leverage them to be successful?**
- **What are your challenges—and how can you combat and overcome any roadblocks?**
- **Are you accountable for your nutrition and exercise?**
- **How is your attitude?**
- **Are you celebrating all your wins?**
- **What does health-style mean for you?**

If you are reading this book, that means that you have committed the next forty-two days (six weeks) to clean eating and a consistent exercise program, which will lead you toward a jump-start to a new health-style path. It takes courage and commitment to make a decision to better your life. One of the most difficult steps to take is often leaving your comfort zone behind, shaking off comfortable old habits, and adopting change. Navigating the process can be daunting at times. There can be ups and downs, roadblocks, and challenges along the way. However, your own intrinsic motivation can help you overcome these obstacles.

This guide will be your constant companion during the next six weeks and will supplement your specific nutrition and fitness plan. The aim of your work within these pages is to connect with your inner power and personal strengths. This guide will also provide with daily accountability for your food and exercise choices via log entries, daily tips and motivation, and positive reinforcement. In the next six weeks, you will explore: nutrition, exercise, accountability, your underlying needs for a new health-style, overcoming roadblocks, celebration and success, long-term lifestyle adoption, and developing your specific health-style goals.

To give you additional support and encouragement, I will also share my own journey with you along the way. But remember: each journey is unique, special, and different than any other. Never compare your own path to any other (even mine). I share my own story simply as assurance that you are not alone in this process.

I am a woman who, like many, many others, has struggled her whole life with fitness and nutrition. I have tried diets and exercise in the past and have yo-yoed my weight up and down and all around. I have recently undergone an intense inward journey, opening myself up to my own new health-style, adopting it for the long term—and losing seventy-five pounds along the way. As you read through my story, I hope you realize that I am sharing my experiences and journey in hopes that they make a positive impact, so that you will continue your own path forward. After all, it took me forty-three years and nearly dying a few times (literally) to connect with my conscious health-style path—and I sincerely wish that no one else has to go through such drastic measures to have their wake-up call.

THE NEXT STEPS ARE COMPLETELY IN YOUR HANDS.

You have the power to change. You have the power to grow and learn. You have the power to succeed.

YOUR PAST DOES NOT DEFINE YOU.

Your past does not lock in your future. You can change your health-style for the better in these moments, no matter where you are coming from.

DO YOU UNDERSTAND THE POWER AND IMPORTANCE IN THOSE IDEAS?

TIME TO GET THIS PARTY STARTED!

HOW TO USE THIS GUIDE

Your journey is only going to be as good and rewarding as the amount of energy and sincere reflection you put into it. A variety of writing techniques can be used when working on the journal pages of this guide, such as: quick bullet points, fragmented sentences, full sentences, and even long diary-like entries. Anything goes—the important thing is that you find a way that works for you—and that you are consistent with it. There are no right or wrong answers or proper writing techniques, since every single person's style is unique.

Extra note pages have been included for you to jot down any comments or notes and can be found at the back of the book for your use.

Throughout, you will be prompted to write your own affirmations (mine are provided as examples). Feel free either to use one that is listed and resonates with you, or to come up with your own. These positive affirmations can motivate and inspire you—as well as to serve as a source of strength on your difficult days. Additionally, on a daily basis you will be asked to write a description of your favorite positive moment from the day. This does not need to be a long entry, and this does not need to be an exercise- or nutrition-related entry. It can be as simple as, "I saw a beautiful sunset." The goal is simply to recognize and record the positive energy surrounding you. I can attest to you that no matter how hard your day is, no matter the challenges or obstacles, there will always be one moment that was better than all the others (even if it is simply the humor in watching a video of a squirrel eating a muffin). Consciously recognizing your affirmations and positive moments will further draw out your inner strengths and make your journey more enjoyable.

Journal entries from my own six-week challenge to jump-start my new healthy way of living are included (**Appendix B**). My personal history describing my own health-style backstory is also covered in pages XXXV–XLII.

WEEKLY FORMAT

Each week of this guide is focused on a separate theme:

- **Week 1: Food and Nutrition**
- **Week 2: Movement and Exercise**
- **Week 3: Goals—What Do You Want?**
- **Week 4: Benefits and Underlying Needs**
- **Week 5: No excuses—What's Stopping You?**
- **Week 6: Designing Your Future—What's Next?**

Within each themed week, the days are broken into the following sections.

At the beginning of each week, you will answer theme-specific questions. I recommend that you *not* work on these out of order (for example, do not skip ahead and work on Week 4 questions before doing Week 1, 2, or 3).

On a daily basis, you should:

1. Log your food and nutrition intake, as well as any applicable supplements taken. (Space is provided to make any notes regarding your meals/snacks, such as: How do you feel at mealtime—tired, hungry, full—and is it difficult to get a meal down? Does the food taste good or bad? Are you trying a new recipe, preparation style, or spice?)

2. Log all exercise activity. (Examples include: specific gym or fitness classes, walking or jogging, swimming or biking, weight training, etc.) Space is provided to make any relevant notes about what you've done.

3. Log your total water intake for the day.

4. Write a description of your favorite positive moment from the day, even though it may have nothing to do with health and wellness. This is a very important daily exercise—*do not skip it!*

At the end of each week, you will be guided to log any Non-Scale Victories (NSV) and Body Measurements. (If you choose, you can also take pictures of yourself.)

GETTING STARTED

Before you start your activity on Monday, Day 1 of 42, you will need to complete the following:

- **Read through Gathering Tools, Statistics and Victories (page XXIII–XXV)**
- **Fill in your Nutrition Accountability Tool (page XXVI)**
- **Fill in your Body Measurements (page XXIX)**
- **Read What Is Your "Why"? (pages XLV–L)**
- **Read Week 1: Food and Nutrition, and complete the week 1 questions (pages 1–8)**

I deserve **HEALTH.**

I deserve **A STRONG BODY.**

I will **BE CHALLENGED.**

I will **NOT GIVE UP.**

I will **OVERCOME.**

I am **UNIQUE.**

I am **NOT ALONE.**

I have **STRENGTH.**

I have **DETERMINATION.**

I choose **MY PATH.**

I can **DO THIS!**

Write your own affirmation:
(You can choose one from above or something new. Write anything that is
meaningful and inspirational for you.)

GOT HEALTH-STYLE?

GATHERING TOOLS, STATISTICS, AND VICTORIES

Positive attitude, accountability, and a solid nutrition and exercise plan are your primary tools for this journey. You will find that it is easier to build momentum and a positive environment when your victories are acknowledged and celebrated. Do not ignore any of your progress or any wins (whether they are tangible or not). Quantifiable body measurements and weight tracking, along with non-quantifiable Non-Scale Victories (NSV) and photographs, are excellent measures of progress, success, and accountability.

Keep in mind that your goals are *your* goals. Some people may want to achieve 8% body fat, while others want to achieve 25% body fat. Some may want an athletic, muscular build, while others want a softer, curvaceous build. Some may want to run a marathon, while others want to walk a 5K. There is no right goal. There is no wrong goal. Your fitness goal is your fitness goal. Embrace it. Own it. Track it. *Do it.*

This guide will supplement *your* specific nutrition plan for *your* specific goals. For example, nutrition plans can vary depending on the goals of your journey: you may want to lose twenty pounds of fat or gain ten pounds of muscle—or you may specifically desire to lower your overall body fat percentage while gaining muscle. Or you may have a totally different goal in mind. Every possible goal will require a tailored food and exercise program. No matter the goal or nutrition plan defining your six-week journey, you can and will connect with your inner power and personal strengths, as well as being accountable for your specific nutrition and exercise program.

The basis for a solid, healthy nutrition plan—no matter your goal—can be achieved by a clean eating regimen, which your gym, doctor, club, or nutritionist may recommend for a health and wellness program. "Clean eating" is a lifestyle of healthy eating, which focuses on using whole, natural, unprocessed, and unrefined foods. A balance of healthy proteins, complex carbohydrates, fresh vegetables and fruits, and healthy fats is utilized. One way to think of clean eating is that you should be able to pronounce all of the ingredients in what you eat: there should be no chemicals, additives, or processed foods that strip away your food's nutritional value.

Some examples of healthy proteins, complex carbohydrates, fresh vegetables, and healthy fats are listed below—but this is (obviously) not a complete list. Your training goals will dictate which specific items you should allow in your nutrition plan.

Healthy Proteins:
Egg Whites, Turkey Breast, White Fish (such as Tilapia, Cod, Halibut), Chicken Breast, Lean Beef, Salmon, Buffalo

Complex Carbohydrates:
Quinoa, Yam, Sweet Potato, Brown Rice, Ezekiel Bread, Steel-Cut Oats, Amaranth

Fresh Vegetables:
Broccoli, Spinach, Kale, Asparagus, Mushrooms, Brussels Sprouts, Collard Greens, Zucchini, Celery, Cauliflower, Peppers, Tomato, Oinons

Healthy Fats:
Avocado, Olive Oil, Coconut Oil, Almond Butter, Ghee, Nuts

If you're just starting out with clean eating, and have heard horror stories, don't worry! Clean eating does not have to be bland and distasteful. It can be flavorful and full of life. Myriad choices of zero-calorie, sugar-free dry spices, mixes, and herbs are waiting for you to explore. Whole aisles can be dedicated to these in the grocery store. Use the list below as a resource as you start exploring the world of flavor. (And remember: many more options are available that are not listed here.)

The Basics:
Rosemary, Dill, Tarragon, Cilantro, Basil, Chervil, Oregano, Mint, Parsley, Thyme, Garlic Powder, Lemon Pepper, Sage, Fennel, Black or Red Pepper

Additional Flare:
Red Curry Powder, Madras Curry Powder, Cumin, Garam Masala, Turmeric, Vindaloo Curry Powder, Coriander, Sumac, Crushed Lemon Omani, Baharat

Extra Depth of Flavor:
Celery Seed, Powdered Onion, Mustard Seed, Lemon Peel, Lavender Pepper, Lavender, Orange Peel, Yellow Mustard

Earthy Tones:

Nutmeg, Cloves, Ginger, Allspice, Pumpkin Pie Spice, Cinnamon, Cardamom, Mace

Spicy:

Ancho Chili Pepper, Chipotle Chili Pepper, Paprika, Smoked Paprika, Sweet Paprika, Wasabi Powder, Mexican-Style Chili Powder, Red Chili Pepper, Chili Powder

To gather more tools to support your health-style journey, consider joining groups around town such as walking groups, running groups, hiking groups, cooking groups, etc. Not sure where to find them? Fitness-related groups can usually be found associated with a local gym.

Explore local seminars, presentations, and informational sessions on topics that further interest you as you undertake this six-week journey. Everyone has different interests. Why not learn all you can about yours? Your local library, bulletin boards at local sports stores, and local newspapers are all great sources to find these activities. Additionally, support groups, seminar schedules, and information on walking/running races, etc., can be found online through websites offering connections in many cities such as: Meetup (www.meetup.com); Active.com (www.active.com); Facebook; and many more.

NUTRITION ACCOUNTABILITY TOOL

What you eat will depend on what your goals are. Hold yourself accountable for *your* specific nutrition plan during these next six weeks and list all your food sources including any possible supplements. Use this list as your grocery list. Keep it simple and you will succeed.

Once you create this list, if an item is not listed here, do not try to justify eating it. Be strong. Be patient. This journey will not happen overnight, but it will happen.

MY NUTRITION DURING THE NEXT 42 DAYS
Remember: If it's not on this list, don't eat it. It's that simple!

CARBOHYDRATES I WILL EAT:

PROTEINS I WILL EAT:

VEGETABLES/FRUIT I WILL EAT:

ANY HEALTHY FATS I WILL EAT:

ANY APPROPRIATE SUPPLEMENTS I WILL TAKE:

HOW MUCH WATER I WILL DRINK EACH DAY:

MARY'S SAMPLE NUTRITION ACCOUNTABILITY TOOL

Below is my own six-week clean eating food list, which was recommended by my gym for my own weight loss program. If an item was not on this list, I simply did not eat it during those six weeks. The point of this list is truly that straightforward.

MY NUTRITION DURING THE NEXT 42 DAYS
Remember: If it's not on this list, don't eat it. It's that simple!

CARBOHYDRATES I WILL EAT:

Quinoa, Yam, Brown Rice, Sweet Potato

PROTEINS I WILL EAT:

Egg Whites, Tilapia, Turkey Breast (no skin), 99% Lean Ground Turkey

VEGETABLES/FRUIT I WILL EAT:

Brussels Sprouts, Spinach, Celery, Green Beans

ANY HEALTHY FATS I WILL EAT:

No fats except Essential Fatty Acids (EFAs) supplements (since these are not produced by the body)

ANY APPROPRIATE SUPPLEMENTS I WILL TAKE:

100% Whey Protein Powder (extra protein source), Glutamine (to aid muscle recovery from workouts), Essential Fatty Acids (EFAs)

HOW MUCH WATER I WILL DRINK EACH DAY:

1 to 2 Gallons per day (128 ounces = 1 Gallon = 16 cups)

BODY MEASURMENTS

Follow your plan. Your body will change. Trust the process.

There will be many reasons to celebrate during the next six weeks. The changes in your body will be one of them. Use a soft tape measure (and the diagram below as a guide) to track and record your starting inches on the next page. Then, as you work through the next six weeks, you can track your measurements and easily see the changes you are making to your body.

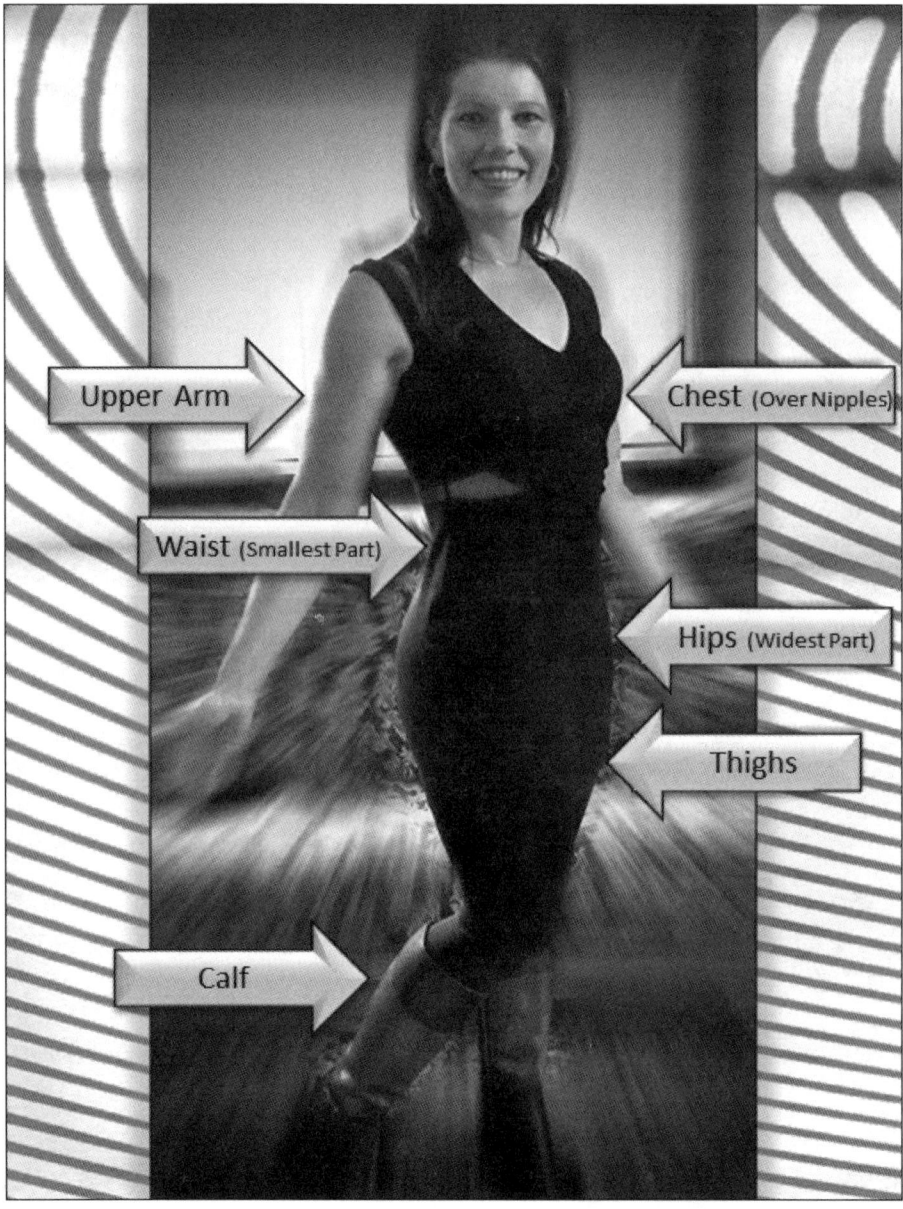

BODY MEASURMENTS

MEASURE YOURSELF. CELEBRATE INCHES.

STARTING MEASUREMENTS

UPPER ARM	CHEST	WAIST	HIPS	THIGHS	CALF

WEEK 1 MEASUREMENTS

UPPER ARM	CHEST	WAIST	HIPS	THIGHS	CALF

WEEK 2 MEASUREMENTS

UPPER ARM	CHEST	WAIST	HIPS	THIGHS	CALF

WEEK 3 MEASUREMENTS

UPPER ARM	CHEST	WAIST	HIPS	THIGHS	CALF

WEEK 4 MEASUREMENTS

UPPER ARM	CHEST	WAIST	HIPS	THIGHS	CALF

WEEK 5 MEASUREMENTS

UPPER ARM	CHEST	WAIST	HIPS	THIGHS	CALF

WEEK 6 MEASUREMENTS

UPPER ARM	CHEST	WAIST	HIPS	THIGHS	CALF

NON-SCALE VICTORIES

Your journey will not be reflected solely in one specific endpoint. Many meaningful milestones will be achieved in the process—and they'll have nothing to do with your bathroom scale. Did your blood pressure go down? Are your clothes fitting looser? Did someone give you a compliment? Can you do a specific physical activity better than before? Did you emotionally overcome a challenge? (There are more examples included on the next page.) Write your Non-Scale Victories (NSVs) down. Honor the wins.

CELEBRATE AND ACKNOWLEDGE ALL FORMS OF VICTORY!

WEEK 1 NSV:

WEEK 2 NSV:

WEEK 3 NSV:

WEEK 4 NSV:

WEEK 5 NSV:

WEEK 6 NSV:

EXAMPLES OF NON-SCALE VICTORIES

This list is a sample of many possibilities of what you might consider to be your Non-Scale Victories (NSVs). You may not experience all of these, and you may have NSVs that are not listed here, since we all have our own goals and lives. Recognize your own victories. NSVs are significant landmarks along your journey.

- **Decreased blood pressure**
- **Stabilized insulin levels**
- **Had a great doctor visit**
- **No longer need medication**
- **Clothes are fitting looser**
- **Needed to tighten belt a notch**
- **Can fit into clothes that I couldn't before**
- **Overcame a temptation**
- **Broke an old habit**
- **Surrounded myself with positivity**
- **Could do a physical activity better than before**
- **Jogged a distance never done before**
- **Mastered a new gym move**
- **Did a full pushup**
- **Increased weights at the gym**
- **Received a compliment**
- **Noticed new muscles**
- **Felt more energized**
- **Played at the park with kids**
- **Was able to attend school functions**
- **Cooked a healthy meal**
- **Housework was easier to do**
- **Yardwork was easier to do**
- **Made it to the gym when I really didn't feel like it**
- **Stuck to my nutrition plan when I really didn't feel like it**

WEIGHT GOAL

Follow your plan. Your body will change. Trust the process.

Weight loss (or muscle weight gain) is not a linear process. Your weight can fluctuate throughout the week—and even throughout the same day. Weight fluctuations are normal. Understand that. Accept it. Water retention, hormonal changes, menstrual cycle, irregular bowel movements, and excess salt intake are all contributing factors to weight fluctuations. Save yourself a lot of anxiety and stay *off* the scale between weigh-ins, as stress can actually slow down weight loss by increasing production of some hormones. Only weigh yourself once a week on your weigh-in day.

Each person loses weight and inches differently and at varying rates based on her specific metabolism and body. Your body will transform under its own guidelines. Be patient. Remain positive. And—whatever you do—do not use your weight as your only defining metric—only consider it along with your body measurements, Non-Scale Victories, and obvious visual changes.

GOAL WEIGHT: ☐

WEEK 1 - START WEIGHT: ☐

WEEK 2 - MONDAY, DAY 08, WEIGHT: ☐

WEEK 3 - MONDAY, DAY 15, WEIGHT: ☐

WEEK 4 - MONDAY, DAY 22, WEIGHT: ☐

WEEK 5 - MONDAY, DAY 29, WEIGHT: ☐

WEEK 6 - MONDAY, DAY 36, WEIGHT: ☐

END WEIGHT: ☐

I will **MOVE FORWARD.**

I will **SUCCEED.**

I will **BE CHALLENGED.**

I will **PERSERVERE.**

I am **DEDICATED.**

I am **COMMITTED.**

I am **STRONG.**

I choose **MY HEALTH-STYLE.**

I choose **TO LIVE NOW.**

I choose **TO BE AWARE OF THE PRESENT.**

I choose **TO DO THIS!**

Write your own affirmation:
(You can choose one from above or something new. Write anything that is meaningful and inspirational for you.)

MARY'S HEALTH-STYLE BACKSTORY

My name is Mary and I am forty-three years young at the time of writing this. I eat clean and exercise on a routine basis. After losing seventy-five pounds, my weight, health status, body mass index (BMI), and body fat composition are well within normal ranges. However, I have not always been this way. In fact, until recently, I had struggled with my health-style for my entire adult life. Here is my story:

Over the years, my weight severely fluctuated, going up and down by eighty or more pounds—from a clothing size eighteen/twenty to a size twelve, and even once to a size ten. I became an expert at selecting good "cover-up" clothing to hide my weight fluctuations as I could not keep any weight off for more than two months at a time.

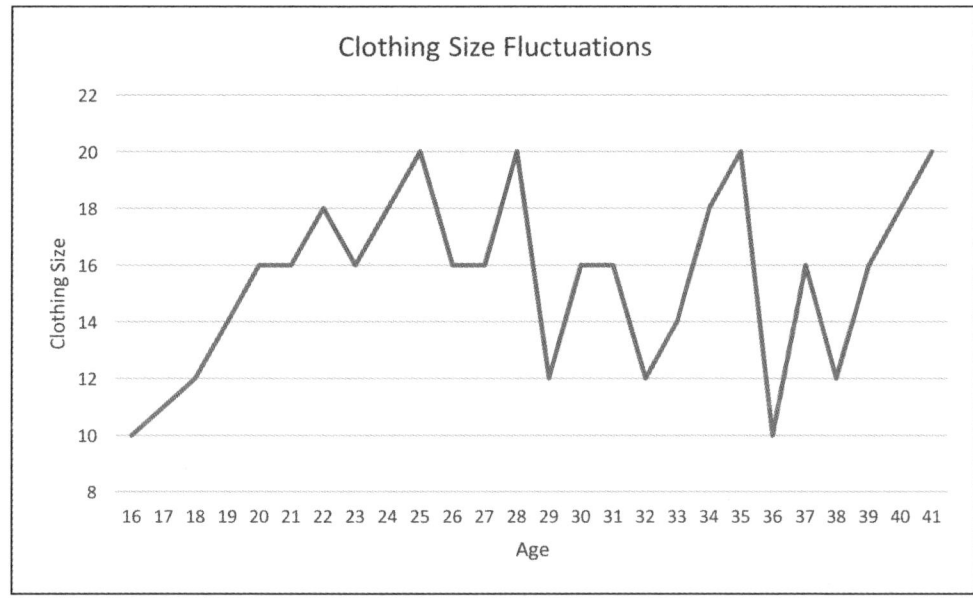

It seems like I tried every diet and exercise program out there. I used special no/low carbohydrate-based cookbooks, ate supplied pre-made foods, drank weight-loss shakes, attempted point systems, and watched video tapes and DVDs galore. Exercise programs started and stopped. Gym memberships were never used. I would lose weight, then slowly (or sometimes very quickly) gain it back again—and then some.

When it came to health and fitness, I did not feel good about myself. I did not understand why I could not manage this area of my life. Where was my motivation? Why could I be successful in other aspects of my life (such as my career), yet be so utterly lost when it came to my health-style?

Every time I gained weight, the extra weight made an impact on the quality of my life, however I was not consciously aware of the dangerous cycle that I was on. I would tell myself that I was built "strong, like mountain folk"—embracing my "big-boned" German/Russian heritage. Physical activities would come in spurts throughout my adult years. At times, I could be the strong girl who could carry her own fifty-pound backpack and hike with her husband, or go on long bike rides of thirty to fifty miles.

During the "lighter" times, I was more active. During the "heavier" times, I struggled to find joy in physical endeavors. For example, back in 2003, surrounded by stunning views and gorgeous scenery during a Hawaiian vacation, I simply wanted to sit in the hotel room. I was out of shape, huffing and puffing—with sore legs and body—through volcanic craters, to pretty waterfalls, and even to a green sand beach. The extra weight contributed to me being physically tired, so we did not make it to many excursions, both because of my limited physical abilities—and my poor attitude. (I did not realize at the time that my poor attitude was a direct result of my poor physical health.)

As my weight fluctuated up and down, I began to lose more and more of myself. I was not consciously aware of any changes to my quality of life. In fact, I focused my attentions "outward," moving from one academic or career goal to another, moving from one task to another, and taking care of clients and management over and over. I defined my own self-worth by outward accomplishments: degrees, titles, labels. I became a workaholic: I had to make another business deal; had to keep getting promoted; had to take care of everything and everybody; had to try to be perfect in everything that I did. I could not show any weakness or vulnerability.

I was mentally strong and successful in my career. I mentored others. Friends and employees came to me for advice. Yet, I had no time to breathe. I felt overwhelmed whenever I slowed down. I just *had* to keep moving in that frenetic fashion since I knew no other way to live. What was I running from? I did not know at the time. It would take me months to schedule a get-together with a friend, I would miss most school functions with my son because I "had" to work, I would put my husband on the back burner and my clients first in order to get the next career goal accomplished. I rarely noticed myself in the mirror and I could not even imagine my own face or recognize myself in photographs. I was living like a "mental zombie"—just going through the motions.

Everything *should have* changed when I was diagnosed with lupus (technically "SLE": Systemic lupus Erythematosus) when I was thirty-five years old. Even so, that diagnosis did not shake me enough to get off the unhealthy cycle that I was on. Instead, because I had struggled for twelve years with various health issues related to lupus prior to my diagnosis. I was simply relieved that I finally knew what was wrong with my health. However, I found that I could not tell anyone that I had lupus. To my workaholic mindset, I couldn't dare be perceived as weak. I did not want special treatment. I did not want extra judgment. I did not want my career held back. I did not want to be seen as anything less than the strong superwoman persona I had created. What would happen to my career if anyone knew I had such a disease? What would people think of me if they knew? I refused to be judged.

Unfortunately, lupus is a chronic autoimmune disease in which the body's immunity attacks itself. You know how you feel when you get the flu with full-body joint pain and severe fatigue? That feeling is what lupus feels like for me when it flares. It attacks my joints (with rheumatoid arthritis and osteoarthritis), as well as my guts/intestines (severe colitis—think Crohn's disease), and includes a few skin issues and chronic fatigue.

My rheumatologist told me to slow down and start taking care of myself (translation: "start living a new health-style path"). I ignored his warnings, telling myself I did not have time for diet and exercise. In 2011, when I was thirty-nine years old, he wrote me a prescription for "Exercise program: Daily." Realizing he was serious, I exercised for a few months and then slipped back into my old habits as I began to feel that the extra activity was taking away too much time from my work efforts. I had other priorities. I had career goals. I continued to define myself by my career. I felt I had something to prove. The doctors gave me steroids and chemotherapy drugs to decrease my immune function, along with injections and pills to treat the lupus. For the rest of the world I put on a show that made everything appear "normal." It was pretty rough behind the scenes. Sometimes, I would have to pull my car over to the side of the road to vomit before a client meeting, as the drugs wreaked havoc on my system. With all this, I still was not consciously ready to change my path.

I had become accustomed to living with health challenges. As a young child, I suffered severe hearing loss, leaving me with 15% hearing capability, so I learned how to read lips. After ear surgery (when I was seven years old), I was able to hear the television, the radio, chirping birds, and the tick-tock of my Mickey Mouse watch for the very first time.

As a toddler, I was diagnosed with Hypoglycemia and would cycle between being nearly comatose and having severe "hyper" fits—until cane sugar was removed from my diet. It seemed like I was always going to the doctor's office for blood tests and the like. I hated it so much that it would take at least four people to hold me down to get a blood sample. Luckily, I acquired a better tolerance to sugar in my teen years (although I still have some issues with it).

At eleven years old, I had a massive brain injury that resulted in epilepsy. It took ten years of brain scans and medications for me to somewhat recover. I also had to re-train my brain and re-learn many language skills and concepts along the way. As a result of that severe injury, I was not allowed to participate in physical education courses at school. No sports. No locker rooms. No team play. Instead, I got extra time to pursue academics, which was just as well, since my brain processed information "differently"—most likely due to the injury. I decided that I just needed to work harder to prove myself. Soon, I found that I was always proving myself. Always proving my self-worth. Always proving my very right to existence.

My first wake-up call came in March 2013, when I was forty-one years old. I was at the height of my career and I delivered a motivational transformation speech to our organization, called "Transforming yourself and your business." Many colleagues told me my talk made a significant positive impact on them. It felt great to be validated, as well as to motivate others. However, no one knew that I was very sick and had been losing physical strength over the past twelve months. I was in a constant state of fatigue and pain and got through my workday out of sheer brute force and caffeine. At first, after work in the evenings I would go straight to the couch to gather energy, but then I started spending all weekend in bed. Eventually it was all I could do to pull myself out of bed for Monday's early-morning conference calls.

A few short weeks after my speech in March 2013, the fatigue and pain became too much to handle and I scheduled an emergency appointment with the rheumatologist on a Wednesday. I was in tears from severe depression; I had felt sick and tired for a year, but it had been taken up a notch—I was in so much pain, all over my body, that I was chronically fatigued and exhausted. My doctor said the inflammation and immune response would progress into organ damage/failure resulting in death if I did not take medical leave immediately; I had to slow down and take care of myself (as I had been told many times before). My immediate reaction was to spend all of the next day working. I did not talk to my management about medical leave until two days later—on a Friday afternoon. I just could not let go. I was trying to figure out how to keep working; how to keep on that path. It was hard to admit that I could not do my job. It was even harder to realize that I could not handle my health.

Three months of emergency medical leave started immediately. I hurt. I was completely drained. It was all I could do to move and function. I was on bed rest. Instead of embracing the change and focusing on recovery, I felt like I had lost all control. I had no power. About two months into my medical leave, I finally consciously connected with my wake-up call.

In my weakened state, I had fallen to the floor and could not lift myself back up. I lay on the carpet, unable to move, and literally had my life flash before me. I was so weak, and I felt like I could die. My husband had to drag me into an upright position and help me back into bed. I finally realized that I needed to change my path. I needed to start to think about my health needs.

Rather than extending medical leave to six months, I gave notice to my employer that I would not be returning to work. I explained that I was going to take time to focus on my health and recovery. It was one of the most difficult decisions that I have ever made.

It was a tough road to recovery. I spent the early summer regaining my strength after months of bed rest. I was up to a clothing size eighteen to twenty again and I could not walk very far due to general weakness, extra weight, and muscle atrophy caused by my lack of movement over time. My son and I took neighborhood walks and gradually worked our way up to a few miles. It was a tough process—our first walk was only to the mailbox and back—but I was determined to regain my energy and life spark. However, I noticed that as I moved more and more, my right knee began to hurt *more and more*.

In late summer, it was discovered that I had a benign tumor inside my knee joint, which literally "blew the joint up" from the inside out. It was severely painful. I found myself back on bed rest, which this time was followed by surgery, rehabilitation, and physical therapy. I had to redo all my efforts again just to walk in the neighborhood. By late fall, I was finally back to moving a few miles. At the time, I decided that 2013 just was not my year.

In November of 2013, after various tests, the rheumatologist formally labeled the lupus as being in remission. It had been a long eight-month battle. However, I was elated. I was making a comeback and I could walk again! I was going to get my life back.

I was so excited that I immediately called my father from the parking lot of the doctor's office to share the good news. As I talked with my dad, only twenty minutes post-appointment, my primary doctor called. I hung up the cell phone on my dad and answered the other line. The doctor informed me that the routine mammogram I had received had come back positive and that I needed to schedule a biopsy and other tests. On December 20, 2013, I was diagnosed with breast cancer.

My heart sank. I was starting to take care of myself for the first time in my life. And this is my reward? Cancer? I had started eating a healthy anti-inflammatory diet a few months prior to help battle the lupus inflammation. I was walking for some exercise. How could cancer possibly happen to me? It was not fair. I became scared and depressed. I withdrew. I tried to pretend everything was all right. I turned to honey-laden peanut butter. I turned to tortilla chips. I cried and cried, and cried some more. My weight shot up to 225 pounds—on my five-foot, six-inch-tall body. Again, I felt helpless and powerless.

My health battle was only beginning. In January 2014, a lumpectomy was performed, along with the axillary lymph nodes being removed. A large section (the size of two decks of cards) was taken out of my breast, and an incision was made along my armpit to remove the lymph nodes, both of which severely affected the mobility of my arm and chest. When the test results came back, I had more bad news: the pathology showed my cancer was not fully removed. I was not cancer free.

In March of 2014, just one year after initiating the lupus battle and medical leave from work, I underwent *three* surgeries to battle cancer. Both ovaries were removed to deplete my body of estrogen, a hormone which had fed the cancer. I had a mastectomy to remove the cancerous breast. The cancer was fully removed. I was cancer free.

However, my body rebelled after I underwent a very complicated and intense "TRAM Flap" procedure to begin my breast reconstruction. My abdomen had to be cut up and guts "rearranged," and I developed colitis as a result. I had massive fatigue. My doctors suspected lupus-related complications. They even suspected pneumonia-related complications.

I was immediately thrown into full-blown menopause with severe hot flashes and sweats. I was so weak that I could not physically move. I ended up in the critical care unit of our hospital for three days before being transferred to the "general" hospital for a week. I was informed that, in short, at any time I could die .

I felt like I was given a choice to simply drift off or stay and fight another day. Part of me wanted to drift off and end it all. I was so weak and tired. I was fed up with the struggle. A larger part of me did not want to leave my son and husband. My boy needed his mama. He had been my coach throughout the lupus recovery and I could not let my coach down. He was counting on me to beat this, so I chose to stay and fight.

I ended up living in the hospital rehabilitation unit for almost another four weeks. I had to relearn everything: how to sit up, to put on shoes, to use a wheelchair, to use a walker, to walk, to go to the bathroom, to take a shower, to brush my teeth, and even to comb my hair.

I had no strength or mobility at first. Eventually, with a lot of hard work, I managed to walk out of the hospital. After the following months of rehabilitation I was walking in the neighborhood again, along with being able to move my arms. It took *so much* work to just be able to lift my arms into the air that I had to celebrate that victory!

In August of 2014, I had another reconstruction surgery across my chest on both sides. It was another small setback in terms of recovery, since I had to start all over again at working to be able to lift my arms into the air. But I was becoming a pro at rehabilitation, making a comeback, and regaining my strength.

During the cancer surgery period and subsequent rehabilitations, I had consciously started thinking about my eating habits. As a result of cutting out gluten, dairy, soy, and cane sugar (in other words, following an anti-inflammatory diet), I had helped conquer the lupus flare-ups and kept it in remission—for the most part. I was determined to do everything in my power to help battle cancer and prevent it from coming back as well.

I quit coffee (I had been up to six or eight cups a day). I quit eating most processed foods. I quit eating foods with added chemicals. I quit drinking wine, whiskey, and most liqueurs. I ended up losing thirty-five pounds through a combination of conscious eating and rehabilitation exercises. I loved the feeling of gaining strength.

I began to feel an inner power I had never known before. I realized that I had felt power in my past career and academic pursuits, but I had never experienced a sense of physical power *in my body*. I became determined to get a strong body so that my cancer would not come back, and so that my lupus would not come back. It was time to get my ass in gear and figure out how to become physically, mentally, and spiritually healthy. I had finally *completely* woken up to my need for a new health-style.

In early October 2014, less than six weeks after my second reconstruction surgery, I decided to embark on a formal exercise program to further my strength and weight-loss efforts. I had developed the endurance to walk ten miles by that point and could lift my arms straight into the air holding three-pound weights. There were still a lot of physical things I could not do like a "normal person," but I had come quite a long way.

I saw an advertisement for a new local gym called "The Camp Transformation Center," which was offering a free program to lose twenty pounds in six weeks through clean eating and exercise. I was the *very first* person to walk through the gym door and sign up for the "6-Week Challenge." The owners, Sam Bakhtiar and Alejandro Font, believed that I could be successful in the program even after I told them of my history, and they made me feel incredibly welcome in the gym.

The day after I signed up at the gym, I started "Shaun T's T25 (by Beachbody)" exercise program in order to get a further jump start on my strength and endurance, since the gym would not open for a few months. For the first time in my life, I completed an entire exercise program! I was mentally committed to a better health-style.

The Camp Transformation Center formally opened on January 19, 2015. I lost twenty-six additional pounds during the 6-Week Challenge. I learned more about clean eating, the different values of food, and what to look for in nutrition labels. I learned about HIIT (High Intensity Interval Training) workouts, weight training, different forms of cardio, and various ways of stretching my muscles.

I also *learned* a lot about myself as part of an intense inward journey. I continued my personal journey and began to connect with my inner motivation, and my true underlying needs and wants. I started to heal old wounds from my past, and began to find peace within. I started reading books, blogs, and magazines, taking courses on fitness and nutrition, having long discussions with trainers, rehabilitation specialists, doctors, and anyone who would give me an ear to discuss health and wellness.

After my six weeks, I continued on with my gym and lost additional weight, bringing my total weight loss to seventy-five pounds (at the time of writing this guide) and to a clothing size of *four*. I continue with my strength and endurance training and have set many short-term and long-term goals for the year to come.

Even so, I know that my journey will continue, since this is my own personal long-term health-style. The journey will never be over. I will always have a healthy goal and a healthy win to look forward to!

My past **DOES NOT DEFINE MY FUTURE!**

I am **UNIQUE.**

I am **SPECIAL.**

I am **NOT ALONE.**

I am **NOT WEAK.**

I will **COMMIT.**

I will **LIVE.**

I will **BE AWARE OF THE PRESENT.**

I choose **MY PATH.**

I choose **TO BE HEALTHY.**

I choose **MY DESIRES.**

Write your own affirmation:
(You can choose one from above or something new. Write anything that is meaningful and inspirational for you.)

WHAT IS YOUR WHY?

"If you always put limit(s) on everything you do, physical or anything else, it will spread into your work and into your life. There are no limits. There are only plateaus, and you must not stay there, you must go beyond them."
- Bruce Lee

"He who has a why to live for can bear almost any how."
- Friedrich Nietzsche

Think about where you are right now—today. Think about where you have been in your life thus far. What is your "why?" that is, why are you embarking upon this six-week journey now? What do you want to accomplish? Why do you want change? Why do you want a new health-style? Has anything stopped you before from adopting a healthy fitness and nutrition lifestyle? Why? Do you have anything standing in your way stopping you right now from getting to where you want to be? What drives you? What motivates you? What strengths do you have to help you get through these next forty-two days?

These are all very important questions for establishing your baseline. Adopting a new health-style is not an easy process. You will probably be pushed emotionally, physically, and mentally. When the journey gets tough, when you want to quit, when you just want to give in, you will need to remind yourself of your "why?"

On the other hand, the process can be rewarding and inspirational. You will learn and grow and discover whole new dimensions of yourself. The answers to "what is your why?" can drive you. These answers will inspire you forward. These answers will motivate you. These answers will continue to empower you. These answers will ultimately fuel your fire and release your inner "roar."

Dig deep. It is time to get to know your internal power.

What do you want to accomplish in the next six weeks?

(For Mary's journal entry, see Appendix B)

_____

Why do you want a new health-style?

(For Mary's journal entry, see Appendix B)

_____

What has stopped you before (what were your previous roadblocks)?

(For Mary's journal entry, see Appendix B)

_____

How will you overcome your roadblock(s) in the next six weeks?

(For Mary's journal entry, see Appendix B)

_____

What strengths do you have, which will enable you to reach your goal? (One way to consider this question is to imagine a previous success in any aspect of your life and draw upon what worked to make it successful.)

(For Mary's journal entry, see Appendix B)

_____

I deserve **A HEALTHY BODY.**

I deserve **HAPPINESS.**

I deserve **PEACE.**

I will **BE CHALLENGED.**

I will **HURT.**

I will **CRY.**

I will **OVERCOME.**

I am **STRONG.**

I am **DETERMINED.**

I can **DO THIS.**

I CAN ***DO THIS!***

_____   _____

Write your own affirmation:
(You can choose one from above or something new. Write anything that is meaningful and inspirational for you.)

WEEK 1: FOOD AND NUTRITION

"Let food be thy medicine and let medicine be thy food."
- Hippocrates

"Food is the most widely abused anti-anxiety drug in America, and exercise is the most potent yet underutilized antidepressant."
- Bill Phillips

The beginning of this journey can be challenging as it takes time and commitment for your body to adjust to a new style of eating. Remember: you and your body *deserve* to be healthy. Your old habits were not working for you, were they? Fight through your inner cravings, as you crave the unhealthy foods that you are trying to rid your body of. You will be forming long-term healthy habits by eating 100% clean during the next six weeks. You are stronger than you think you are!

Both proper diet and exercise are imperative for your health-style success. The old adage "you are what you eat" is true. "Abs are made in the kitchen" is also true. Nutrition and any applicable supplements are key to supporting your journey.

Nutrition is crucial to your metabolism. What is your metabolism? "Metabolism" can be summed up as a step-wise process by which your body converts what you eat and drink into the energy your body needs to operate. The key feeders of your metabolism come in the forms of: protein, carbohydrates, fat, and water. In fancy terms, metabolism is described by two categories: catabolism (the breakdown of nutrients to release energy) and anabolism (the building and repair of tissues, which consumes energy).

Proteins are found in every single cell in our body and are the primary building blocks of our muscles, heart, organs, tissues, bone, skin, and hair. They are made up of tiny units called amino acids. Our body cannot make all the different kinds of amino acids needed to build a protein, and therefore we must get these essential amino acids from the foods we eat.

Carbohydrates in food come in three forms: sugar, starch, and fiber. Simple carbohydrates (sugars) supply a quick release of energy and are described as "fast carbs." These are found in refined and processed foods, cane sugar, fruits, jams, honey, maple syrup, agave, and most soda. Complex carbohydrates (starches) supply a slower, sustained release of energy and are described as "slow carbs." Examples of complex carbohydrates include: green vegetables, starchy vegetables like yam and sweet potato, beans, legumes, and whole grains.

Simple carbohydrates/fast carbs can disrupt your metabolism and cause weight gain, obesity, type 2 diabetes, and cardiovascular disease if they are eaten on a routine basis. The slow release of energy by complex carbohydrates/slow carbs is key to sustaining a healthy diet, and can assist with weight loss (when combined with steady exercise).

Fiber is also an important part of a healthy diet and plays a critical role in proper digestion. It is found in vegetables, grains, and fruit. Why is digestion important? A study published in *Nature Reviews Immunology*[1] showed that maintaining digestive health is imperative to the body's overall well-being. In fact, 70% of the body's immune system resides in the gastrointestinal tract and a malfunction here can lead to autoimmune disease, allergies, and cancer. Fiber moves through the GI tract to remove waste and toxins that your body does not need, helps feed the important bacteria in the gut and contribute to GI health, aids regular bowel movements, and helps absorb nutrients by slowing digestion so the body has more time to take in any important nutrients.

Many important *Fats* (healthy fats) are meaningful to your metabolism because they help absorb soluble vitamins (vitamins A, D, E). Examples of healthy fats include: avocado, olive oil, coconut oil, almond butter, and ghee. Essential fats cannot be made by the body and must be taken in through diet or supplements. These essential unsaturated fats (essential fatty acids) play many important roles, including aiding in: muscle formation, fat-loss, immune function, and hair and skin health. Saturated fats (unhealthy fats) are found in meat and dairy products and examples include the fats found in: fatty beef, chicken with skin, cream, ice cream, butter, and cheese. The American Heart Association has shown that saturated fats and trans-fats (and cholesterol) have been linked to heart disease and arteriosclerosis.[2] According to the Mayo Clinic, trans-fats can actually *double* your chances of heart disease.[3] Yet, these fats are found in *most*

---

[1]   J. L. Round and S. K. Mazmanian, "The gut microbiota shapes intestinal immune responses during health and disease," *Nature Reviews Immunology* 9 (2009): 313-323.

[2]   Joseph Alpert, "What Diet Should We Recommend for Our Patients?" *Circulation* (2011), http://circ.ahajournals.org/content/124/10/e258.full, accessed May 19, 2016.

[3]   "Trans fat is double trouble for your heart health," Mayo Clinic website (June 19, 2015), http://www.mayoclinic.org/trans-fat/art-20046114, accessed May 19, 2016.

ready-made foods, chips, bakery items with long shelf lives, fried foods, creamers and margarine, and many more things. If you're not sure whether these are in what you're eating, simply read your food labels.

Water is imperative to your nutrition and body's metabolism because it is used in most bodily functions including the healthy maintenance of your cells, tissues, and organs. Sixty to eighty percent of your body is composed of water, which can aid in fat loss, proper circulation, the removal of toxins from the digestive tract, and suppression of your appetite. A study published in the journal *Obesity* showed that absolute and relative increases in drinking water were associated with significant loss of body weight and fat over time by lowering total energy intake and altering metabolism.[4] Basically, staying properly hydrated allows the body to have more energy and burn fat. How much water does it take to stay properly hydrated? This depends on many factors, such as: how active you are, your training goals, your health, and where you live. In general, The Institute of Medicine recommend three liters (0.8 gallons) per day[5], and The International Sports Sciences Association recommends twelve glasses (0.76 gallons) per day[6], while health and fitness programs could increase recommendations to one to two gallons per day to account for increased physical activities and water loss through sweat and respiration. However much water you choose to drink, make sure to have consistent access to it throughout the day. Hydration will be a key component to your success.

A clean-eating food plan involving healthy proteins, complex carbohydrates, fresh vegetables, healthy fats, and proper hydration can ramp up your metabolism. A clean-eating regimen encourages you to eat five or six meals spread throughout the day, which can aid with portion control by alleviating hunger, which could otherwise lead to overeating. In general, we as a nation are eating too much because food portions are out of control. A study conducted back in 2002 by the Department of Nutrition and Food Studies at New York University showed that marketplace food portions have progressively grown in size since the 1970s, and have continued in parallel with the US obesity epidemic[7].

To aid your portion control, you can measure and weigh food to stay on track. One method of measurement involves counting caloric and macronutrient (protein, carbohydrate, fat) intake, but this is not a practical method for the everyday person. On the other hand, weighing food with a food-grade scale is an excellent way to get acquainted with proper portion sizes. For example, in general a woman's meal portion

---

4   J. D. Stookey, et al, "Drinking water is associated with weight loss in overweight dieting women independent of diet and activity," *Obesity* 16, no. 11 (2008): 2481-2488.

5   "Dietary Reference Intakes: Water, Potassium, Sodium, Chloride, and Sulfate," The National Academies of Sciences, Engineering, and Medicine–Health and Medicine Division website (released February 11, 2004), http://www.nationalacademies.org/hmd/Reports/2004/Dietary-Reference-Intakes-Water-Potassium-Sodium-Chloride-and-Sulfate.aspx, accessed May 23, 2016.

6   http://www.issaonline.edu/.

7   L. R. Young, et al, "The Contribution of Expanding Portion Sizes to the US Obesity Epidemic," *The American Journal of Public Health* 92, no. 2 (2002): 246-249.

consists of two ounces of complex carbohydrates and four ounces of healthy protein, while a man's portion consists of three ounces of complex carbohydrates and six ounces of healthy protein. Some meal plans consider unlimited quantities of vegetables in a clean-eating regimen, while other plans and goals require portioning of the vegetables in order to keep track of the specific macronutrients consumed. An alternative "hand method" is described on a serving size card by the National Heart, Lung, and Blood Institute: a serving of carbohydrates (such as sweet potato) is the size of a fist, and a serving of protein is the size of a deck of cards (or an opened hand).[8] Additionally, portion control plates and containers can be found in the marketplace. As you make your decisions, pick a portion measurement style that will be realistic for you to maintain while still holding yourself accountable.

Meal preparation and planning will be a key strategy to your nutrition success. Consider the following questions:

- What are you going to eat today?
- What will you eat this week?
- How will you stay hydrated?
- Are you going out to a restaurant? If so, can you study the menu beforehand so you know how to stay on track?
- Will your work cater food sometime this week and will you need to bring in your own meal instead?
- Are you going to be stuck somewhere, and do you have a snack or meal to tide you over?
- Do you have time to cook every night?
- Should you prepare multiple meals at one time so you can "grab and go"?

Once you have a plan in place, you can be prepared for any unplanned scenarios. You can do this!

---

8   "Serving Size Portions," National Heart, Lung, and Blood Institute website (September 30, 2013), http://www.nhlbi.nih.gov/health/educational/wecan/eat-right/distortion.htm, accessed May 23, 2016.

WHAT IS YOUR RELATIONSHIP WITH NUTRITION?

What factors influenced your food choices before starting this six-week journey? Do stress or emotions typically influence your choices? Describe them and how they do so.

(For Mary's journal entry, see Appendix B)

What are the biggest nutritional challenges for you and your family?

(For Mary's journal entry, see Appendix B)

_____

Have you ever considered the nutritional value of food when making food choices? Why or why not?

How did you hydrate before starting this program (how much and what kinds of liquid did you drink everyday)? Would you like to make changes to that pattern?

(For Mary's journal entry, see Appendix B)

_____

How will you hold yourself accountable for your food choices during the next six weeks?

(For Mary's journal entry, see Appendix B)

_____

THIS IS MONDAY, DAY 1. Let's double check the completion of your activities. Put a checkmark next to each item you've completed.

_____ **Read "Gathering Tools, Statistics and Victories"** *p. XXIII*

_____ **Filled in your Nutrition Tool List** *p. XXVI*

_____ **Filled in your Start Measurements** *p. XXIX*

_____ **Took your Picture** *(if you chose)*

_____ **Filled in your Goal Weight** *p. XXXII*

_____ **Filled in your Start Weight** *p. XXXII*

_____ **Read "What Is Your Why?** *p. XLV*

_____ **Answered the questions in "What Is Your Why?"** *p. XLVI*

_____ **Read "Week 1: Food and Nutrition"** *p. 1*

_____ **Answered the questions in "What Is Your Relationship With Nutrition?"** *p. 5*

MARY'S EXAMPLE DAILY LOG ENTRY *Day 1/42*

IT'S ONLY SIX WEEKS.

MEAL	TIME	WHAT DID YOU EAT? (INCLUDE ANY APPLICABLE SUPPLEMENTS)	NOTES*
BREAKFAST	7:30	4 oz. egg whites and spinach for omelet, 2 oz. sweet potato	*I like egg whites from the carton!*
SNACK	10:00	1 Scoop chocolate protein powder with Glutamine	*Love this protein powder*
LUNCH	12:30	4 oz. 99% lean ground turkey, Brussels sprouts, 2 oz. brown rice	*Seems like a lot of food here*
SNACK	3:00	1 Scoop chocolate protein powder with Glutamine	*Tastes like a shake*
DINNER	6:00	4 oz. tilapia, spinach, and celery mix, 2 oz. quinoa	*Quinoa wasn't bad. May try adding some spices next time.*
SNACK	8:30	1 Scoop chocolate protein powder with EFAs	*Feels like dessert. Am I eating too much?*

*Examples: How do you feel? Did the food taste good or bad?
Was it a new recipe, preparation style, or spice? Any other comments.

HOW MUCH WATER DID I HAVE TODAY?
Remember: 128 ounces = 1 gallon = 16 cups = a well hydrated body

1 Gallon. This seems like a ton of water!!! I peed all day long!

EXERCISE ACTIVITY	TIME SPENT	NOTES*
Camp Class. Arm day.	*55 minutes*	*Warm up was very tough. A lot of cardio. Had to do a lot of modifications.*
Neighborhood walk.	*40 minutes*	*Walked to the school with my son today. It was tough getting up the hill!*

*Examples: How do you feel? Was an activity easy or challenging? Did you gain any strength or endurance? Any other comments.

WRITE A DESCRIPTION OF YOUR FAVORITE POSITIVE MOMENT FROM TODAY:
Remember: It's up to you to create your positive environment and draw out your inner strength. Recognize any positivity surrounding you. Find it. Create it. Celebrate it. Daily.

This evening, I walked to the school and back with my son for a neighborhood stroll. We took the "hilly way." I had to stop and rest a couple of times, but I made it up the hill! It was awesome to do that hill with him. On the way home we saw some gorgeous colors in the sky for a beautiful sunset. I love this time of year when the colors in the sky are so vibrant. Put me in a great mood for the evening.

THIS IS MONDAY, DAY 1. Welcome to the next six weeks! Congratulations for taking the first steps toward your new health-style. It's time to eat clean, exercise, and hydrate properly. This is the time to dig deep and find your inner power. Game on. You can do this! IT'S ONLY SIX WEEKS.

MEAL	TIME	WHAT DID YOU EAT? (INCLUDE ANY APPLICABLE SUPPLEMENTS)	NOTES*
BREAKFAST			
SNACK			
LUNCH			
SNACK			
DINNER			
SNACK			

*Examples: How do you feel? Did the food taste good or bad?
Was it a new recipe, preparation style, or spice? Any other comments.

HOW MUCH WATER DID I HAVE TODAY?
Remember: 128 ounces = 1 gallon = 16 cups = a well hydrated body

EXERCISE ACTIVITY	TIME SPENT	NOTES*

*Examples: How do you feel? Was an activity easy or challenging? Did you gain any strength or endurance?
Any other comments.

WRITE A DESCRIPTION OF YOUR FAVORITE POSITIVE MOMENT FROM TODAY:
Remember: It's up to you to create your positive environment and draw out your inner strength. Recognize any positivity surrounding you. Find it. Create it. Celebrate it. Daily.

FOOD PREPARATION is key. Think "Grab and Go." Do not set up to get off track. Have a plan in place. Carry food/snacks with you as needed. Cook your meals in bulk and measure the portions. Store in zipper-seal bags, airtight containers, or other carry containers. It is very easy to eat healthy as long as you are prepared for it.

MAKE A LIFESTYLE CHANGE!

MEAL	TIME	WHAT DID YOU EAT? (INCLUDE ANY APPLICABLE SUPPLEMENTS)	NOTES*
BREAKFAST			
SNACK			
LUNCH			
SNACK			
DINNER			
SNACK			

*Examples: How do you feel? Did the food taste good or bad?
Was it a new recipe, preparation style, or spice? Any other comments.

HOW MUCH WATER DID I HAVE TODAY?
Remember: 128 ounces = 1 gallon = 16 cups = a well hydrated body

EXERCISE ACTIVITY	TIME SPENT	NOTES*

*Examples: How do you feel? Was an activity easy or challenging? Did you gain any strength or endurance?
Any other comments.

WRITE A DESCRIPTION OF YOUR FAVORITE POSITIVE MOMENT FROM TODAY:
Remember: It's up to you to create your positive environment and draw out your inner strength. Recognize any positivity surrounding you. Find it. Create it. Celebrate it. Daily.

DAILY LOG ENTRY

Day 3/42

IT TAKES WORK to reset your metabolism. Give your body time to acclimate. You may be feeling nauseated as your body is detoxing from the sugar, preservatives, and processed foods you ate before. This feeling is normal and will subide. Trust the process and trust clean eating.

IT WILL GET BETTER.

MEAL	TIME	WHAT DID YOU EAT? (INCLUDE ANY APPLICABLE SUPPLEMENTS)	NOTES*
BREAKFAST			
SNACK			
LUNCH			
SNACK			
DINNER			
SNACK			

*Examples: How do you feel? Did the food taste good or bad?
Was it a new recipe, preparation style, or spice? Any other comments.

HOW MUCH WATER DID I HAVE TODAY?
Remember: 128 ounces = 1 gallon = 16 cups = a well hydrated body

EXERCISE ACTIVITY	TIME SPENT	NOTES*

*Examples: How do you feel? Was an activity easy or challenging? Did you gain any strength or endurance? Any other comments.

WRITE A DESCRIPTION OF YOUR FAVORITE POSITIVE MOMENT FROM TODAY:
Remember: It's up to you to create your positive environment and draw out your inner strength. Recognize any positivity surrounding you. Find it. Create it. Celebrate it. Daily.

Day 4/42

PROPER HYDRATION allows the body to have more energy and burn more fat. Drinking about a gallon of water per day can be challenging. Drink throughout the day (do not guzzle your water all at once). Perhaps add lemon, cucumber, or fresh mint for flavoring. Take a water bottle with you everywhere you go.

JUST KEEP GOING. BELIEVE!

MEAL	TIME	WHAT DID YOU EAT? (INCLUDE ANY APPLICABLE SUPPLEMENTS)	NOTES*
BREAKFAST			
SNACK			
LUNCH			
SNACK			
DINNER			
SNACK			

*Examples: How do you feel? Did the food taste good or bad?
Was it a new recipe, preparation style, or spice? Any other comments.

HOW MUCH WATER DID I HAVE TODAY?
Remember: 128 ounces = 1 gallon = 16 cups = a well hydrated body

EXERCISE ACTIVITY	TIME SPENT	NOTES*

*Examples: How do you feel? Was an activity easy or challenging? Did you gain any strength or endurance?
Any other comments.

WRITE A DESCRIPTION OF YOUR FAVORITE POSITIVE MOMENT FROM TODAY:
**Remember: It's up to you to create your positive environment and draw out your inner
strength. Recognize any positivity surrounding you. Find it. Create it. Celebrate it. Daily.**

Day 5 /42

THE WEEKEND is almost here. It can be easy to get out of your routine or distracted and forget your path on weekends. Do not sabotage your hard work and go off track. Have a weekend plan in place before you go to bed tonight. When will you meal prep? What will you do for exercise this weekend?

YOU WILL BE SUCCESSFUL.

MEAL	TIME	WHAT DID YOU EAT? (INCLUDE ANY APPLICABLE SUPPLEMENTS)	NOTES*
BREAKFAST			
SNACK			
LUNCH			
SNACK			
DINNER			
SNACK			

*Examples: How do you feel? Did the food taste good or bad?
Was it a new recipe, preparation style, or spice? Any other comments.

HOW MUCH WATER DID I HAVE TODAY?
Remember: 128 ounces = 1 gallon = 16 cups = a well hydrated body

EXERCISE ACTIVITY	TIME SPENT	NOTES*

*Examples: How do you feel? Was an activity easy or challenging? Did you gain any strength or endurance? Any other comments.

WRITE A DESCRIPTION OF YOUR FAVORITE POSITIVE MOMENT FROM TODAY:
Remember: It's up to you to create your positive environment and draw out your inner strength. Recognize any positivity surrounding you. Find it. Create it. Celebrate it. Daily.

DAILY LOG ENTRY

Day 6 / 42

IS YOUR FOOD TASTING BLAND?

Discover new flavors! Check out the spice aisle in your local grocer, spice shop, or farmer's market to explore new flavors and ideas. Do you like savory? Spicy? Earthy? Blends? There are many possibilities of zero-calorie, sugar-free dry spices and herbs out there. Have fun with your food.

STAY CLEAN. DON'T CHEAT!

MEAL	TIME	WHAT DID YOU EAT? (INCLUDE ANY APPLICABLE SUPPLEMENTS)	NOTES*
BREAKFAST			
SNACK			
LUNCH			
SNACK			
DINNER			
SNACK			

*Examples: How do you feel? Did the food taste good or bad?
Was it a new recipe, preparation style, or spice? Any other comments.

HOW MUCH WATER DID I HAVE TODAY?
Remember: 128 ounces = 1 gallon = 16 cups = a well hydrated body

EXERCISE ACTIVITY	TIME SPENT	NOTES*

*Examples: How do you feel? Was an activity easy or challenging? Did you gain any strength or endurance? Any other comments.

WRITE A DESCRIPTION OF YOUR FAVORITE POSITIVE MOMENT FROM TODAY:
Remember: It's up to you to create your positive environment and draw out your inner strength. Recognize any positivity surrounding you. Find it. Create it. Celebrate it. Daily.

Day 7/42

TAKE TIME TODAY to reflect on any Non-Scale Victories from the week. (p. XXX). Take and record your body measurements. (p. XXIX). If you choose, also take pictures of yourself (front view, side view, back view). You and your journey are much more than a simple number on the scale.

FOOD PREP IS VITAL.

MEAL	TIME	WHAT DID YOU EAT? (INCLUDE ANY APPLICABLE SUPPLEMENTS)	NOTES*
BREAKFAST			
SNACK			
LUNCH			
SNACK			
DINNER			
SNACK			

*Examples: How do you feel? Did the food taste good or bad?
Was it a new recipe, preparation style, or spice? Any other comments.

HOW MUCH WATER DID I HAVE TODAY?
Remember: 128 ounces = 1 gallon = 16 cups = a well hydrated body

EXERCISE ACTIVITY	TIME SPENT	NOTES*

*Examples: How do you feel? Was an activity easy or challenging? Did you gain any strength or endurance?
Any other comments.

WRITE A DESCRIPTION OF YOUR FAVORITE POSITIVE MOMENT FROM TODAY:
Remember: It's up to you to create your positive environment and draw out your inner strength. Recognize any positivity surrounding you. Find it. Create it. Celebrate it. Daily.

It is **ALRIGHT TO FEEL.**

It is **ALRIGHT TO CRY.**

It is **ALRIGHT TO BE ANGRY.**

I can **CRAVE OLD HABITS.**

I can **LOOK FOR EXCUSES.**

I will **NOT GIVE IN.**

I will **NOT GIVE UP.**

I am **RESILIENT.**

I am **TOUGH.**

I choose **TO LIVE NOW.**

I choose **MY PATH.**

Write your own affirmation:
(You can choose one from above or something new. Write anything that is
meaningful and inspirational for you.)

WEEK 2: MOVEMENT AND EXERCISE

"If it doesn't challenge you, it won't change you."

"It does not matter how slow you go—so long as you do not stop."
– Confucius

Exercise may be one of the best things for a successful health-style. There are health risks of unfitness (such as increased risk of chronic disease) as well as many benefits of fitness (exercise can increase energy, improve mood and self-esteem, help with weight loss and curb appetite, strengthen muscles, tone body, improve balance and coordination, keep bones strong, change your health for the better, reduce your risk of chronic disease, build a stronger immune system, and even give you better sleep patterns). Many who live a clean-eating lifestyle exercise five to six times per week. The discipline and consistency of committing to an exercise program can bleed over into other aspects of life, leaving participants healthy, happy, and full of energy!

Moderate exercise is safe for most people. However, according to the President's Council on Physical Fitness and Sports, a physician should be consulted prior to beginning an exercise program if you have or ever had: high blood pressure; heart trouble; risk factors for heart attack or stroke (like a family history of problems or high cholesterol, or if you smoke); dizzy spells; diabetes (because increased exercise can affect insulin needs); arthritis or other bone and joint problems that could limit physical activities; severe muscular, ligament, or tendon problems; back problems; or other known medical conditions.[1] Also seek appropriate medical attention for any injury prior to taking on an exercise program. Do not be afraid to use any applicable wraps, braces, or sports tapes to support an injury and assist in healing during your fitness program. Additionally, you should be sure to modify your exercises to address any physical limitations.

---

1   "Physical Activity Guidelines for Americans," President's Council on Fitness, Sports & Nutrition website, http://www.fitness.gov/be-active/physical-activity-guidelines-for-americans/, accessed May 23, 2016.

Patience is a prerequisite when starting a new exercise program. *Go at your own pace.* Remember: it does not matter what physical accomplishments any other person can do. It does not matter what physical accomplishments you achieved last year, five years ago, or twenty years ago. What matters is *you*—today. What can you do today? How can you keep up the hard work and dedication and do a little bit better tomorrow? When you think you cannot push any more, push a little harder. If you cannot finish a routine today, then plan to go a few minutes longer tomorrow. You will be surprised by what you are capable of with slow and steady improvements in strength, endurance, and range of motion. Small, attainable goals are key. Setting mini milestones for yourself will keep pushing you forward.

Ask yourself during the weeks to come, "What can I do today that I could not do on Day 1?"—and make note of those victories.

Most people benefit from a healthy mix of many elements of exercise. Strength training through lifting free weights and/or using resistance bands and machines is important for muscle and bone strength—as well as increasing speed. Stability and balance training can support your core body strength. Flexibility and stretching enhance the range of motion of your joints, stretch and strengthen muscles, and help prevent muscle strains and soft tissue injury. An increase in flexibility can also improve balance and coordination. Aerobic exercise can build endurance, strengthen your heart and lungs, burn fat, aid with weight loss, and increase your cardiorespiratory endurance (breathing).

Muscle soreness is a common by-product of pushing your body to its limits and can be challenging when starting a new fitness program. Don't worry—some muscle pain is normal. All people, even those who have been exercising for years, get sore and experience discomfort. Generally, the pain and stiffness felt in muscles occurs beginning anywhere from several hours up to three days after a workout in people who are unaccustomed to strenuous exercise. Do your best to push through the soreness, and it will begin to fade more quickly once your body adapts to your new exercise routine and intensity. Soreness will stay around longer with infrequent training as it will take longer for your body to adapt, so consistency is key. At the same time, it is important to note: you should be careful not to over-train. You will need a rest day each week. Even professional athletes take a rest day to allow the body time to recover from the strain on muscles, tendons, ligaments, bones, and joints.

At the same time, not all muscle pain is created equally. You will need to pay attention to your body and understand the difference between a good hurt (soreness, or a "dull ache" in a muscle or joint) and a bad hurt (injury, or a deep, sharp and pulling pain in a very specific spot). Many people do not understand the difference and simply give up on a new exercise program as the result of feeling a "common, good hurt." It should be obvious, of course, that for any "bad hurt," you should promptly seek medical attention.

Treating and recovering from soreness might include using foam rollers, stretching, taking Epsom salt baths, and hydrating. Foam roller exercises and stretching are a great way to release any muscle tightness (the fancy term for this is "self-myofascial release"), increase blood flow to the muscles, aid muscle repair, decrease recovery time, and increase your range of motion by lengthening and elongating muscles. Ideas for foam roller and stretching exercises can be easily obtained on the Internet and are often found in books and fitness magazines. Stretching throughout the day can also greatly aid recovery from muscle soreness and pain. Epsom salt (the common name for magnesium sulfate) baths can be beneficial in the treatment of sore muscles as well (simply add one or two cups of the salts to a warm, forty-minute bath). And remember that proper hydration will make a huge difference for you as water makes up 65–75% of muscle weight and is critical for muscle tissue recovery and growth.

Sleep is the most important time of day for a body to recover and is integral for optimal muscle recovery, repair, and growth. The food and nutrients we consume throughout the day are used to replace energy and rebuild muscle during sleep. Guidelines by the National Sleep Foundation recommend at least seven hours of sleep per night. We all know that it can be difficult to get a solid night's sleep between work schedules, family responsibilities, school schedules, and many other life-related tasks. Some tips for getting a good night's sleep suggested by the National Sleep Foundation include: going to sleep and waking up at the same time every day, avoiding naps, controlling exposure to bright light within two hours of your bedtime, getting exercise, and being smart about what—and when—you eat and drink (stay away from caffeine, alcohol, cigarettes, and heavy meals before bed).[2]

No matter what happens in your first days of exercise, do *not* quit before you have given yourself the chance to experience the benefits of exercise and improved fitness. Too tired? Too sore? Now is not the time for excuses. You have committed six weeks to changing your life. You can get this done. Not enough time? It is important to schedule your fitness routine for a time when there is little chance of being interrupted by other life responsibilities such as your family, school, or job. Have a plan. Schedule your workouts on the calendar like any other appointments. Lay out your workout clothes the night before, or leave a gym bag in the car. Exercise needs to become part of your daily routine for a lifetime of health and wellness. This is your journey now.

---

2   "How Much Sleep Do We Really Need?" National Sleep Foundation website, https://sleepfoundation.org/how-sleep-works/how-much-sleep-do-we-really-need, accessed May 23, 2016.

WHAT IS YOUR VIEW ON EXERCISE?

Have you tried (and given up on) an exercise program before starting this health-style program? What are your reasons for not starting or continuing with that past fitness program?

(For Mary's journal entry, see Appendix B)

What are the strengths you can use to combat any barriers to exercise?
(For Mary's journal entry, see Appendix B)

As you start you new path, describe your health and emotional benefits from doing an exercise program.

(For Mary's journal entry, see Appendix B)

_____

Describe your current consistency with a workout program.

(For Mary's journal entry, see Appendix B)

_____

Describe any social support that will hold you accountable to your new exercise program. How will _you_ hold yourself accountable?

(For Mary's journal entry, see Appendix B)

_____

Real life adventures!
What would you do?

Consider this scenario:

You have a friend named Joe who has high blood pressure, who joined a six-week exercise program and lost fifteen pounds. During those six weeks Joe was able to talk to his doctor and stop taking his medication as his blood pressure moved back into the normal range. As the weeks went on, Joe decided that he did not like to get up early for his workouts because he was too busy at work. Joe began to make excuses and stopped his exercise program at the gym where he is still a member. Through your encouragement, he agrees to meet you at the gym but does not show up.

What advice would you give Joe?

_____

THIS IS MONDAY, DAY 8. Let's double check the completion of your activities. Put a checkmark next to each item you've completed.

_____ **Logged a Daily Positive Moment for Week 1**

_____ **Logged a Daily Meal, Hydration, and Exercise Plan for Week 1**

_____ **Filled in your Body Measurments for Week 1** *p. XXIX*

_____ **Listed your Non-Scale Victories for Week 1** *p. XXX*

_____ **Filled in your Monday, Day 08, Weight** *p. XXXII*

_____ **Took applicable pictures for Week 1 (if you chose)**

_____ **Read "Week 2: Movement and Exercise"** *p. 29*

_____ **Answered the questions in "What Is Your View on Exercise?"** *p. 33*

_____ **Answered the questions in "What Would You Do?"** *p. 38*

THIS IS YOUR JOURNEY. Do not directly compare your journey to anyone else's. Your body is your body. Your story is your story. You are unique. You are special. You are you. Your body will transform in its own time. Some people see measurable results sooner and some see them later. Be patient. Trust this process.

LISTEN TO YOUR BODY.

MEAL	TIME	WHAT DID YOU EAT? (INCLUDE ANY APPLICABLE SUPPLEMENTS)	NOTES*
BREAKFAST			
SNACK			
LUNCH			
SNACK			
DINNER			
SNACK			

*Examples: How do you feel? Did the food taste good or bad?
Was it a new recipe, preparation style, or spice? Any other comments.

HOW MUCH WATER DID I HAVE TODAY?
Remember: 128 ounces = 1 gallon = 16 cups = a well hydrated body

EXERCISE ACTIVITY	TIME SPENT	NOTES*

*Examples: How do you feel? Was an activity easy or challenging? Did you gain any strength or endurance?
Any other comments.

WRITE A DESCRIPTION OF YOUR FAVORITE POSITIVE MOMENT FROM TODAY:
Remember: It's up to you to create your positive environment and draw out your inner strength. Recognize any positivity surrounding you. Find it. Create it. Celebrate it. Daily.

THE PROPER FITTING SHOE can make all the difference. Before you begin running, go to a sport-running store and have a store clerk look at the way you walk. Select the best support for your feet and gait. The support and balance you will receive from your shoes varies across brands and styles. One brand does not work for everyone, and choosing the right brand will (literally) propel you forward. GIVE IT YOUR ALL!

MEAL	TIME	WHAT DID YOU EAT? (INCLUDE ANY APPLICABLE SUPPLEMENTS)	NOTES*
BREAKFAST			
SNACK			
LUNCH			
SNACK			
DINNER			
SNACK			

*Examples: How do you feel? Did the food taste good or bad?
Was it a new recipe, preparation style, or spice? Any other comments.

HOW MUCH WATER DID I HAVE TODAY?
Remember: 128 ounces = 1 gallon = 16 cups = a well hydrated body

EXERCISE ACTIVITY	TIME SPENT	NOTES*

*Examples: How do you feel? Was an activity easy or challenging? Did you gain any strength or endurance? Any other comments.

WRITE A DESCRIPTION OF YOUR FAVORITE POSITIVE MOMENT FROM TODAY:
Remember: It's up to you to create your positive environment and draw out your inner strength. Recognize any positivity surrounding you. Find it. Create it. Celebrate it. Daily.

DAILY LOG ENTRY

If you experience an injury, do not be afraid to modify any exercises to accommodate your change in abilities. There is almost always a modified move for the knee, ankle, wrists, back, or any other body part. Communicate with your trainer, teacher, coach, or gym facility. If you need to, look into appropriate braces, sports medicine wraps, or kinesiology ("KT") tape for extra support.

IT'S OKAY TO CRY!

MEAL	TIME	WHAT DID YOU EAT? (INCLUDE ANY APPLICABLE SUPPLEMENTS)	NOTES*
BREAKFAST			
SNACK			
LUNCH			
SNACK			
DINNER			
SNACK			

*Examples: How do you feel? Did the food taste good or bad?
Was it a new recipe, preparation style, or spice? Any other comments.

HOW MUCH WATER DID I HAVE TODAY?
Remember: 128 ounces = 1 gallon = 16 cups = a well hydrated body

EXERCISE ACTIVITY	TIME SPENT	NOTES*

*Examples: How do you feel? Was an activity easy or challenging? Did you gain any strength or endurance? Any other comments.

WRITE A DESCRIPTION OF YOUR FAVORITE POSITIVE MOMENT FROM TODAY:
Remember: It's up to you to create your positive environment and draw out your inner strength. Recognize any positivity surrounding you. Find it. Create it. Celebrate it. Daily.

EVERYONE WHO TRAINS experiences soreness. Seek medical attention for any sharp or tearing pain, but otherwise work through the aches. Stretch to relieve sore muscles. Use a foam roller or a recovery supplement such as glutamine. Take Epsom salt baths. Use muscle rubs like Icy Hot, Tiger Balm, or essential oils. You will work past the soreness. You can do this!

YOU DESERVE TO SUCCEED.

MEAL	TIME	WHAT DID YOU EAT? (INCLUDE ANY APPLICABLE SUPPLEMENTS)	NOTES*
BREAKFAST			
SNACK			
LUNCH			
SNACK			
DINNER			
SNACK			

*Examples: How do you feel? Did the food taste good or bad?
Was it a new recipe, preparation style, or spice? Any other comments.

HOW MUCH WATER DID I HAVE TODAY?
Remember: 128 ounces = 1 gallon = 16 cups = a well hydrated body

EXERCISE ACTIVITY	TIME SPENT	NOTES*

*Examples: How do you feel? Was an activity easy or challenging? Did you gain any strength or endurance?
Any other comments.

WRITE A DESCRIPTION OF YOUR FAVORITE POSITIVE MOMENT FROM TODAY:
Remember: It's up to you to create your positive environment and draw out your inner strength. Recognize any positivity surrounding you. Find it. Create it. Celebrate it. Daily.

PUSH YOURSELF and do your best at each workout. Your best is all you can do. Only *you* really know if you are holding back during your exercise program. Can you push harder? Set mini-goals for yourself in the workouts, get to your goal, then set a new goal to work toward. Leave it all in your exercise routine!

NO OBSTACLE IS TOO HARD.

MEAL	TIME	WHAT DID YOU EAT? (INCLUDE ANY APPLICABLE SUPPLEMENTS)	NOTES*
BREAKFAST			
SNACK			
LUNCH			
SNACK			
DINNER			
SNACK			

*Examples: How do you feel? Did the food taste good or bad?
Was it a new recipe, preparation style, or spice? Any other comments.

HOW MUCH WATER DID I HAVE TODAY?
Remember: 128 ounces = 1 gallon = 16 cups = a well hydrated body

EXERCISE ACTIVITY	TIME SPENT	NOTES*

*Examples: How do you feel? Was an activity easy or challenging? Did you gain any strength or endurance? Any other comments.

WRITE A DESCRIPTION OF YOUR FAVORITE POSITIVE MOMENT FROM TODAY:
Remember: It's up to you to create your positive environment and draw out your inner strength. Recognize any positivity surrounding you. Find it. Create it. Celebrate it. Daily.

DAILY LOG ENTRY Day 13/42

THE WEEKEND IS HERE What are you going to do with it? Are you going to stay on your nutrition and fitness plan? Are you getting enough rest? Try to get at least seven hours of sleep each night. Your body needs (and deserves) to recover from all the work you are doing. Take the time to rejuvenate!

DO NOT LOOK BACK!

MEAL	TIME	WHAT DID YOU EAT? (INCLUDE ANY APPLICABLE SUPPLEMENTS)	NOTES*
BREAKFAST			
SNACK			
LUNCH			
SNACK			
DINNER			
SNACK			

*Examples: How do you feel? Did the food taste good or bad?
Was it a new recipe, preparation style, or spice? Any other comments.

HOW MUCH WATER DID I HAVE TODAY?
Remember: 128 ounces = 1 gallon = 16 cups = a well hydrated body

EXERCISE ACTIVITY	TIME SPENT	NOTES*

*Examples: How do you feel? Was an activity easy or challenging? Did you gain any strength or endurance? Any other comments.

WRITE A DESCRIPTION OF YOUR FAVORITE POSITIVE MOMENT FROM TODAY:
Remember: It's up to you to create your positive environment and draw out your inner strength. Recognize any positivity surrounding you. Find it. Create it. Celebrate it. Daily.

DAILY LOG ENTRY *Day* 14/42

CELEBRATE YOURSELF for putting in the effort this week toward a new health-style path. Two weeks down. Woo-hoo! Reflect on your Non-Scale Victories (p.XXX); are you stronger in your workout as compared to Day 01? Remember to take your body measurements (p. XXIX) and pictures of yourself (if you choose).

NEVER DOUBT YOUR ABILITY.

MEAL	TIME	WHAT DID YOU EAT? (INCLUDE ANY APPLICABLE SUPPLEMENTS)	NOTES*
BREAKFAST			
SNACK			
LUNCH			
SNACK			
DINNER			
SNACK			

*Examples: How do you feel? Did the food taste good or bad?
Was it a new recipe, preparation style, or spice? Any other comments.

HOW MUCH WATER DID I HAVE TODAY?
Remember: 128 ounces = 1 gallon = 16 cups = a well hydrated body

EXERCISE ACTIVITY	TIME SPENT	NOTES*

*Examples: How do you feel? Was an activity easy or challenging? Did you gain any strength or endurance?
Any other comments.

WRITE A DESCRIPTION OF YOUR FAVORITE POSITIVE MOMENT FROM TODAY:
Remember: It's up to you to create your positive environment and draw out your inner strength. Recognize any positivity surrounding you. Find it. Create it. Celebrate it. Daily.

I will **BE CHALLENGED.**

I will **LIVE.**

I am not **ALONE.**

I am **DEVOTED.**

I am **SPECIAL.**

I deserve **HEALTH.**

I deserve **A STRONG BODY.**

I can **SUCCEED.**

I choose to **SUCCEED.**

I will **SUCCEED.**

My past **DOES NOT DEFINE MY FUTURE.**

_____ _____

Write your own affirmation:
(You can choose one from above or something new. Write anything that is
meaningful and inspirational for you.)

WEEK 3: GOALS—WHAT DO YOU WANT?

"In my experience . . . achievement depends on willingness to accept a challenge, take risks, make errors and the belief that one has the control over the outcomes. Achievement is hindered by perfectionism, fear of failure, and the belief that control, credit and/or blame belong to someone else."

– P. Theroux

"Setting goals is the first step in turning the invisible into the visible."

– Tony Robbins

Congratulations! You've made it to Week 3. How is it going so far? Do you believe that you can change your health-style for the better? Do you believe that you can reach your goals? It is your choice as to what you imagine this week—and the next three weeks—will be. What do you expect of yourself? Now is the time to further connect with your intentions to take back your internal power. You can make things happen, one step at a time.

The power of your intentions and acting upon them is the "special sauce" to achieving your goals. Dr. Deepak Chopra, describes "intention" as the starting point of every dream.[1] Intention is defined as: the thing that you plan to do or achieve (that is, your aim or purpose).[2] What is your intention? What is your attitude? Do you feel positive? Do you feel negative? Do you feel like you do not care? Do you feel frustrated? Do you feel excited? Where will you put your focus this week?

---

1   Deepak Chopra, "5 Steps to Setting Powerful Intentions," *The Chopra Center*, http://www.chopra.com/ccl/5-steps-to-setting-powerful-intentions, accessed May 19, 2016.

2   http://www.merriam-webster.com/dictionary/intention

Your state of mind and attitude are incredibly important to determining the outcome of this health-style journey. Make sure that you maintain a positive and "present" tone. For example: rather than saying, "I don't want a fat bum and thighs;" I will set my intention as, "I want a healthy, strong, and toned bum and thighs." This more optimistic tone allows me to focus my intention on the positive aspects of becoming healthy and fit, instead of berating myself daily because I am not at my dream goal. Your intentions will become more powerful, stronger, and more achievable when they are driven by positive energy.

Positive self-talk (also known as "inner dialogue") can also make a difference for your journey. Imagine self-talk as having a sports-like commentator inside your head making comments on everything you do—from support and cheerleading to massive criticism. Except, unlike listening to an announcer in an arena or while watching TV, *you* have control over this voice. The manner in which you talk to yourself can have a big influence on how you feel and act, as well as impacting your confidence and self-esteem. A study led by the Institute for the Psychology of Elite Performance found that endurance bikers who used positive self-talk pedaled longer than athletes who did not.[3] Below are just a few examples of ways to turn negative self-talk into alternative, positive approaches.

Negative Self-Talk Versus Alternative Positive Self-Talk

Negative: I didn't go to the gym every day last week. I'm a failure at this exercise program.

Positive Alternative: I went to the gym four times last week and gave it my all. Going to the gym and getting some exercise is a lot better than getting none.

Negative: I didn't follow my food plan at lunch today; I just can't stick with this program.

Positive Alternative: I am embracing new, healthy nutritional habits so well that I now recognize when I go off plan. Healthy food is good for me.

Negative: This traffic has something against me. I was planning on going to the gym today, but I am stuck on the freeway. I just can't win.

Positive Alternative: You never know for certain what will happen with rush hour traffic, so I'm glad I have a plan for doing exercise at home on days that I can't make it in time to the gym.

---

3   A. W. Blanchfield, et al, "Talking yourself out of exhaustion: the effects of self-talk on endurance performance," *Medicine & Science in Sports & Exercise* 46, no. 5 (2014): 998-1007.

As you move toward your health and fitness goals, surround yourself with positive influences. Remove any and all negativity around you, including your own self-thoughts. Shut down any self-doubts. Surround yourself with people who can give you moral support, who inspire and motivate you, who keep you up, and who have your back.

If you have no one in your "positive camp" what can you do to create a positive environment? Some ideas include surrounding yourself with like-minded people at the gym or fitness class who have similar goals, reading motivational books and blogs, or listening to motivational speeches and lectures. Consider moods and feelings to be "contagious." Be mindful as to how you project your own moods and feelings. If you focus on the negative the majority of the time, chances are those around you will also focus on the negative. When you create your space, consider who will be invited to share it.

Look at what you have accomplished in the past two weeks. Can you imagine yourself eating clean and exercising like this two months ago? You are getting physically, mentally, and emotionally stronger every day on this journey. But remember that this journey is not a linear process. Do not get frustrated if your results are not as fast as you would like. It did not take you only two weeks to get into your current shape, so do not expect to achieve your endpoint goals in two weeks either. Be patient and be kind with yourself. It takes courage, strength, and determination to change your life for the better—but I know you can do this. You are doing this one day, one meal, and one workout at a time.

This week, it is time to consider how you look at yourself, your goals, your intent, your personal growth, your wants, your actions—and your journey. This journey is, after all, in your hands.

Choose to go get it!

LET'S DO SOME DIGGING.

Why do you continue to choose a new health-style?

(For Mary's journal entry, see Appendix B)

_____

What is working for you so far in this journey? What isn't working?

(For Mary's journal entry, see Appendix B)

_____

How can you build on—and strengthen—what is working?

(For Mary's journal entry, see Appendix B)

_____

Describe your current state in terms of your feelings and attitude. Are you positive, negative, blah, energetic, tired, scared, happy, wishful, lonely, frustrated, or something else? Get it all out!

(For Mary's journal entry, see Appendix B)

_____

How can you encourage yourself to stay on track with your new health-style?

(For Mary's journal entry, see Appendix B)
_____

Do you believe you can achieve this and, if so, why?

(For Mary's journal entry, see Appendix B)

_____

Are there any demotivating factors or roadblocks currently in your way? If so, what can you do to remove them?

(For Mary's journal entry, see Appendix B)

_____

Real life adventures! What would you do?

Consider this scenario:

You have diligently followed your nutrition program with appropriate meal prep and food guidelines for three weeks. You attend a social function with friends and family. At this function a full buffet of food, including desserts, (none of which is on your plan) is served. Additionally, your friends and family will be drinking wine and beer. You come prepared and bring your own meal in order to keep your intake in line with your goals. Someone close to you begins to tease you for not joining in the buffet and alcohol.

How do you feel when this happens? What do you do? What are your strengths and weaknesses in this scenario?

_____

THIS IS MONDAY, DAY 15. Let's double check the completion of your activities. Put a checkmark next to each item you've completed.

_____ **Logged a Daily Positive Moment for Week 2**

_____ **Logged a Daily Meal, Hydration, and Exercise Plan for Week 2**

_____ **Filled in your Body Measurments for Week 2** *p. XXIX*

_____ **Listed your Non-Scale Victories for Week 2** *p. XXX*

_____ **Filled in your Monday, Day 15, Weight** *p. XXXII*

_____ **Took applicable pictures for Week 2 (if you chose)**

_____ **Read "Week 3: Goals—What Do You Want?"** *p. 57*

_____ **Answered the questions in "Let's Do Some Digging"** *p. 61*

_____ **Answered the questions in "What Would You Do?"** *p. 68*

YOU HAVE MADE THE DECISION to change your life for the better. Remember your goals and do your best. Look at yourself in the mirror tonight and say, "I did the best I could today. I gave it my all." Be true to yourself! Only you know if you are sincerely committed to the process, giving it your all, and following your plan.

IT'S IN THE ATTITUDE.

MEAL	TIME	WHAT DID YOU EAT? (INCLUDE ANY APPLICABLE SUPPLEMENTS)	NOTES*
BREAKFAST			
SNACK			
LUNCH			
SNACK			
DINNER			
SNACK			

*Examples: How do you feel? Did the food taste good or bad?
Was it a new recipe, preparation style, or spice? Any other comments.

HOW MUCH WATER DID I HAVE TODAY?
Remember: 128 ounces = 1 gallon = 16 cups = a well hydrated body

EXERCISE ACTIVITY	TIME SPENT	NOTES*

*Examples: How do you feel? Was an activity easy or challenging? Did you gain any strength or endurance? Any other comments.

WRITE A DESCRIPTION OF YOUR FAVORITE POSITIVE MOMENT FROM TODAY:
Remember: It's up to you to create your positive environment and draw out your inner strength. Recognize any positivity surrounding you. Find it. Create it. Celebrate it. Daily.

EVERY DAY OF EXERCISING, eating clean, and staying hydrated is a win. Your actions make a positive and significant difference in your life. They facilitate your transformation. You are stronger in body and mind. How do you choose to perceive this journey? What is your attitude going to be for the rest of this week?

ALWAYS DO ONE MORE.

MEAL	TIME	WHAT DID YOU EAT? (INCLUDE ANY APPLICABLE SUPPLEMENTS)	NOTES*
BREAKFAST			
SNACK			
LUNCH			
SNACK			
DINNER			
SNACK			

*Examples: How do you feel? Did the food taste good or bad?
Was it a new recipe, preparation style, or spice? Any other comments.

HOW MUCH WATER DID I HAVE TODAY?
Remember: 128 ounces = 1 gallon = 16 cups = a well hydrated body

EXERCISE ACTIVITY	TIME SPENT	NOTES*

*Examples: How do you feel? Was an activity easy or challenging? Did you gain any strength or endurance? Any other comments.

WRITE A DESCRIPTION OF YOUR FAVORITE POSITIVE MOMENT FROM TODAY:
Remember: It's up to you to create your positive environment and draw out your inner strength. Recognize any positivity surrounding you. Find it. Create it. Celebrate it. Daily.

REMIND YOURSELF why you started this journey. What is your "why?" (pp. XLV–L). Reflect on your accomplishments thus far. Hold your head high and embrace your inner confidence. You have come so far. You have the courage to break old habits and embrace a new path. You have the strength to keep going.

MAKE A LIFESTYLE CHANGE!

MEAL	TIME	WHAT DID YOU EAT? (INCLUDE ANY APPLICABLE SUPPLEMENTS)	NOTES*
BREAKFAST			
SNACK			
LUNCH			
SNACK			
DINNER			
SNACK			

*Examples: How do you feel? Did the food taste good or bad?
Was it a new recipe, preparation style, or spice? Any other comments.

HOW MUCH WATER DID I HAVE TODAY?
Remember: 128 ounces = 1 gallon = 16 cups = a well hydrated body

EXERCISE ACTIVITY	TIME SPENT	NOTES*

*Examples: How do you feel? Was an activity easy or challenging? Did you gain any strength or endurance?
Any other comments.

WRITE A DESCRIPTION OF YOUR FAVORITE POSITIVE MOMENT FROM TODAY:
Remember: It's up to you to create your positive environment and draw out your inner strength. Recognize any positivity surrounding you. Find it. Create it. Celebrate it. Daily.

DAILY LOG ENTRY

Day 18/42

KEEP UP A ROUTINE. Practice and discipline is needed to keep a consistent exercise and clean-eating routine. Do you still want this new path as badly as you did when you started? What actions can you take to keep moving forward toward your goals? Your dedication is worth it. You are capable of more than you realize.

TACKLE EACH NEW DAY.

MEAL	TIME	WHAT DID YOU EAT? (INCLUDE ANY APPLICABLE SUPPLEMENTS)	NOTES*
BREAKFAST			
SNACK			
LUNCH			
SNACK			
DINNER			
SNACK			

*Examples: How do you feel? Did the food taste good or bad?
Was it a new recipe, preparation style, or spice? Any other comments.

HOW MUCH WATER DID I HAVE TODAY?
Remember: 128 ounces = 1 gallon = 16 cups = a well hydrated body

EXERCISE ACTIVITY	TIME SPENT	NOTES*

*Examples: How do you feel? Was an activity easy or challenging? Did you gain any strength or endurance? Any other comments.

WRITE A DESCRIPTION OF YOUR FAVORITE POSITIVE MOMENT FROM TODAY:
Remember: It's up to you to create your positive environment and draw out your inner strength. Recognize any positivity surrounding you. Find it. Create it. Celebrate it. Daily.

"OBSTACLES DON'T HAVE TO STOP YOU.

If you run into a wall, don't turn around and give up. Figure out how to climb it, go through it, or work around it" (Michael Jordan). When you get up every morning, tell yourself that you can do this. *You are* doing this! No bump in the road can stop you on your path.

TAKE PRIDE IN PROGRESS!

MEAL	TIME	WHAT DID YOU EAT? (INCLUDE ANY APPLICABLE SUPPLEMENTS)	NOTES*
BREAKFAST			
SNACK			
LUNCH			
SNACK			
DINNER			
SNACK			

*Examples: How do you feel? Did the food taste good or bad?
Was it a new recipe, preparation style, or spice? Any other comments.

HOW MUCH WATER DID I HAVE TODAY?
Remember: 128 ounces = 1 gallon = 16 cups = a well hydrated body

EXERCISE ACTIVITY	TIME SPENT	NOTES*

*Examples: How do you feel? Was an activity easy or challenging? Did you gain any strength or endurance?
Any other comments.

WRITE A DESCRIPTION OF YOUR FAVORITE POSITIVE MOMENT FROM TODAY:
Remember: It's up to you to create your positive environment and draw out your inner strength. Recognize any positivity surrounding you. Find it. Create it. Celebrate it. Daily.

DAILY LOG ENTRY Day 20 / 42

THE WEEKEND IS HERE! Stay strong. How do you choose to live this weekend? Your positive attitude can lead to positive success. What is your intent? What do you want? What actions will you choose to do to keep focused on your goals? This is your weekend. Make the most of it. Have a plan. Stay on track!

STAY FIT. DON'T QUIT.

MEAL	TIME	WHAT DID YOU EAT? (INCLUDE ANY APPLICABLE SUPPLEMENTS)	NOTES*
BREAKFAST			
SNACK			
LUNCH			
SNACK			
DINNER			
SNACK			

*Examples: How do you feel? Did the food taste good or bad?
Was it a new recipe, preparation style, or spice? Any other comments.

HOW MUCH WATER DID I HAVE TODAY?
Remember: 128 ounces = 1 gallon = 16 cups = a well hydrated body

EXERCISE ACTIVITY	TIME SPENT	NOTES*

*Examples: How do you feel? Was an activity easy or challenging? Did you gain any strength or endurance?
Any other comments.

WRITE A DESCRIPTION OF YOUR FAVORITE POSITIVE MOMENT FROM TODAY:
Remember: It's up to you to create your positive environment and draw out your inner strength. Recognize any positivity surrounding you. Find it. Create it. Celebrate it. Daily.

DAILY LOG ENTRY

CAN YOU IMAGINE YOURSELF eating clean and exercising like this three months ago? You are becoming physically, mentally, and emotionally stronger every day of this journey. Celebrate any Non-Scale Victories you experienced this week (p. XXX). Record your body measurements (p. XXIX) and take pictures of yourself (if you choose).

ONE DAY AT A TIME.

MEAL	TIME	WHAT DID YOU EAT? (INCLUDE ANY APPLICABLE SUPPLEMENTS)	NOTES*
BREAKFAST			
SNACK			
LUNCH			
SNACK			
DINNER			
SNACK			

*Examples: How do you feel? Did the food taste good or bad?
Was it a new recipe, preparation style, or spice? Any other comments.

HOW MUCH WATER DID I HAVE TODAY?
Remember: 128 ounces = 1 gallon = 16 cups = a well hydrated body

EXERCISE ACTIVITY	TIME SPENT	NOTES*

*Examples: How do you feel? Was an activity easy or challenging? Did you gain any strength or endurance?
Any other comments.

WRITE A DESCRIPTION OF YOUR FAVORITE POSITIVE MOMENT FROM TODAY:
Remember: It's up to you to create your positive environment and draw out your inner strength. Recognize any positivity surrounding you. Find it. Create it. Celebrate it. Daily.

I choose **MY PATH.**

I choose **TO BE AWARE OF THE PRESENT.**

I can **BREAK OLD HABITS.**

I can **CONQUER ANY EXCUSES.**

I will **BE CHALLENGED.**

I will **PRESERVE.**

I am **DEDICATED.**

I am **COMMITTED.**

I am **STRONG.**

I am **AM ME.**

I can **DO THIS!**

Write your own affirmation:
(You can choose one from above or something new. Write anything that is meaningful and inspirational for you.)

WEEK 4: BENEFITS AND UNDERLYING NEEDS

"Energy and persistence conquer all things."
- **Benjamin Franklin**

"Write your injuries in dust, your benefits in marble."
- **Benjamin Franklin**

"You are what you do, not what you say you'll do."
- **Carl Jung**

Welcome to the halfway point of your six-week adventure! You have now made it through three weeks! Take time to reflect and to praise the inner strength that it took to get here. You are stronger in both body and mind than when you started. You are learning to choose your own path. You are gaining confidence. You are gaining strength. Keep moving forward. Keep digging deeper. Dig deeper in your exercises. Dig deeper in your inward reflection. Dig deeper in your commitment. You are in the process of generating your own new health-style.

The physical benefits of this process may begin to shine through at this point—if they haven't already. Do you feel lighter? Do you feel stronger? Do you have more endurance than you did at this time last month? Are your clothes fitting looser? Can you see more muscle definition? How is your general health? Are you noticing any differences in your blood pressure, cholesterol levels, insulin levels, or patterns of inflammation?

How are you feeling at this point? Can you list any adjectives describing you now that you did not consider at the start of this journey? Here is a list to help you start:

adaptable	dynamic	kind
adventurous	easygoing	optimistic
affectionate	emotional	patient
ambitious	energetic	persistent
brave	enthusiastic	powerful
communicative	fearless	proactive
compassionate	friendly	reliable
considerate	funny	resourceful
courageous	generous	self-confident
creative	hard-working	self-disciplined
decisive	helpful	sincere
determined	independent	tough
diligent	inventive	versatile

Unfortunately, the "honeymoon phase" is over now that you are at the halfway point. No longer is the excitement of trying something new hanging in the air. This means that it is true commitment and decision time. Are you going to throw in the towel and go back to your old habits? Or will you stick with this program to see this to the end and change your health-style for the better? What are the physical and emotional benefits of continuing this adventure and achieving your goals? How can you stay positive and constantly encourage yourself and others to stay on path?

It is possible that your journey may bring up sensitive triggers and/or uncover underlying needs which you never knew you had, and these in turn could bring up reactions based on feelings associated with specific experiences from your past. Stress, anxiety, fear, worry, trauma, and other factors can cause strong reactions. Can you think of a time that you "blew up" in a situation and didn't understand why you had had such a severe reaction? Or have you been stressed out and turned to munching on a big bowl of ice cream or a bag of potato chips—or downed multiple beers—as a result? These are often examples of reacting to a trigger. Look at your own life. How do you react in times of stress? Do you get angry or shut down? Do you get needy or are you a people-pleaser? Do you blame others? Do you turn to food? Do you turn to alcohol? Do you turn to shopping? Every person reacts differently to stressful stimuli based on their own past experiences. What drives you toward a constructive or deconstructive reaction is based in the underlying needs that are important to you—even if you don't consciously recognize them.

Every person has needs. Every person reacts in one way or another when she feels like her needs are not being met. Do you know what your underlying needs are? To get you to start thinking about this question, look at this list of the most common underlying needs compiled by Dr. Marcia Reynolds and see if any resonate with you. Do you have a need for: acceptance, being understood, being in control, attention, peacefulness, order, safety, fun, respect, being needed, being right, comfort, balance, variety, predictability, new challenges, being liked, being valued, being treated fairly, consistency, love, feeling included, or autonomy?[1]

Dig deep and understand your triggers and needs in order to adopt and maintain a long-term healthy lifestyle. Try to learn to accept your feelings so that you are not controlled by them. This is a process. This is a journey. This will not happen overnight. However, you can start down the path of understanding—*now*.

You deserve to be healthy! You deserve to have energy! You deserve to be happy in your health-style!

---

1   Marcia Reynolds, *Outsmart Your Brain! How to Make Success Feel Easy* (Phoenix: Covisioning, 2004): 29.

EXPLORE YOUR BENEFITS

In what way do you measure the quality of your health? In what way do you measure the quality of your life? Are they the same?

(For Mary's journal entry, see Appendix B)

_____

What successes have you had on your journey thus far? What do you envision your future to look like?

(For Mary's journal entry, see Appendix B)

_____

Describe any constructive or destructive behaviors which contribute to your health. Describe any outside influences (such as friends, family, work environment, etc.) which impact your overall health. How do you feel about these behaviors and influences?

(For Mary's journal entry, see Appendix B)

_____

What are some of the underlying needs in your life? Why are these important to you?

(For Mary's journal entry, see Appendix B)

_____

Describe a past situation or experience that, when you think about it, causes old feelings and behaviors to come up. How does this contribute to—or take away from—your current health-style path?

(For Mary's journal entry, see Appendix B)

_____

THIS IS MONDAY, DAY 22. Let's double check the completion of your activities. Put a checkmark next to each item you've completed.

_____ **Logged a Daily Positive Moment for Week 3**

_____ **Logged a Daily Meal, Hydration, and Exercise Plan for Week 3**

_____ **Filled in your Body Measurments for Week 3** *p. XXIX*

_____ **Listed your Non-Scale Victories for Week 3** *p. XXX*

_____ **Filled in your Monday, Day 22, Weight** *p. XXXII*

_____ **Took applicable pictures for Week 3 (if you chose)**

_____ **Read "Week 4: Benefits and Underlying Needs"** *p.87*

_____ **Answered the questions in "Explore Your Benefits"** *p. 91*

CONSIDER THE FREEDOM of choice. Look at what you have chosen to accomplish and learn thus far. No one else did this for you. You now have the choice to go back to your old, unhealthy habits, but you also have the choice to keep moving forward toward a new, healthy lifestyle. This is your choice. What is it going to be? Got health-style?

NO MORE "I CAN'T."

MEAL	TIME	WHAT DID YOU EAT? (INCLUDE ANY APPLICABLE SUPPLEMENTS)	NOTES*
BREAKFAST			
SNACK			
LUNCH			
SNACK			
DINNER			
SNACK			

*Examples: How do you feel? Did the food taste good or bad?
Was it a new recipe, preparation style, or spice? Any other comments.

HOW MUCH WATER DID I HAVE TODAY?
Remember: 128 ounces = 1 gallon = 16 cups = a well hydrated body

EXERCISE ACTIVITY	TIME SPENT	NOTES*

*Examples: How do you feel? Was an activity easy or challenging? Did you gain any strength or endurance? Any other comments.

WRITE A DESCRIPTION OF YOUR FAVORITE POSITIVE MOMENT FROM TODAY:
Remember: It's up to you to create your positive environment and draw out your inner strength. Recognize any positivity surrounding you. Find it. Create it. Celebrate it. Daily.

USE YOUR IMAGINATION and visualize

where you want to be. What does your new healthy lifestyle look like? How do you look? How do your clothes look? How does your family look? How does your kitchen look? How does the refrigerator look? How do your activities look? Keep those images in your mind and see what they will bring you.

STICK WITH THE PROGRAM!

MEAL	TIME	WHAT DID YOU EAT? (INCLUDE ANY APPLICABLE SUPPLEMENTS)	NOTES*
BREAKFAST			
SNACK			
LUNCH			
SNACK			
DINNER			
SNACK			

*Examples: How do you feel? Did the food taste good or bad?
Was it a new recipe, preparation style, or spice? Any other comments.

HOW MUCH WATER DID I HAVE TODAY?
Remember: 128 ounces = 1 gallon = 16 cups = a well hydrated body

EXERCISE ACTIVITY	TIME SPENT	NOTES*

*Examples: How do you feel? Was an activity easy or challenging? Did you gain any strength or endurance?
Any other comments.

WRITE A DESCRIPTION OF YOUR FAVORITE POSITIVE MOMENT FROM TODAY:
Remember: It's up to you to create your positive environment and draw out your inner strength. Recognize any positivity surrounding you. Find it. Create it. Celebrate it. Daily.

CAN YOU SAY "NO"? Get comfortable saying no! Say it out loud: "no, No, NO!" There are times where you need to say no to your friends and family in order to stay on track with your health-style plan, especially within these six weeks. No junk food is worth it. No partying all night is worth it. No alcohol is worth it. *no No NO!*

STAY FOCUSED. PUSH LIMITS.

MEAL	TIME	WHAT DID YOU EAT? (INCLUDE ANY APPLICABLE SUPPLEMENTS)	NOTES*
BREAKFAST			
SNACK			
LUNCH			
SNACK			
DINNER			
SNACK			

*Examples: How do you feel? Did the food taste good or bad?
Was it a new recipe, preparation style, or spice? Any other comments.

HOW MUCH WATER DID I HAVE TODAY?
Remember: 128 ounces = 1 gallon = 16 cups = a well hydrated body

EXERCISE ACTIVITY	TIME SPENT	NOTES*

*Examples: How do you feel? Was an activity easy or challenging? Did you gain any strength or endurance? Any other comments.

WRITE A DESCRIPTION OF YOUR FAVORITE POSITIVE MOMENT FROM TODAY:
Remember: It's up to you to create your positive environment and draw out your inner strength. Recognize any positivity surrounding you. Find it. Create it. Celebrate it. Daily.

WE ALL HAVE STRESS and we all have personal triggers. How do you deal with your stress? Explore creative outlets to release it. Perhaps you could relieve yours by writing in a journal, drawing, working out at the gym extra hard, or simply talking with a friend, family member, or religious leader. Get your stress out in a healthy way. Be prepared for stress so that it doesn't stress you out!

THE CHANGE IS AMAZING!

MEAL	TIME	WHAT DID YOU EAT? (INCLUDE ANY APPLICABLE SUPPLEMENTS)	NOTES*
BREAKFAST			
SNACK			
LUNCH			
SNACK			
DINNER			
SNACK			

*Examples: How do you feel? Did the food taste good or bad?
Was it a new recipe, preparation style, or spice? Any other comments.

HOW MUCH WATER DID I HAVE TODAY?
Remember: 128 ounces = 1 gallon = 16 cups = a well hydrated body

EXERCISE ACTIVITY	TIME SPENT	NOTES*

*Examples: How do you feel? Was an activity easy or challenging? Did you gain any strength or endurance? Any other comments.

WRITE A DESCRIPTION OF YOUR FAVORITE POSITIVE MOMENT FROM TODAY:
Remember: It's up to you to create your positive environment and draw out your inner strength. Recognize any positivity surrounding you. Find it. Create it. Celebrate it. Daily.

DAILY LOG ENTRY   Day 26/42

CAN YOU KEEP YOUR PROMISES?

You made a promise and commitment to yourself to embark on this six-week journey toward a new healthy lifestyle. Are you thinking of breaking your promise? Do you have any doubts? Challenges are difficult. If it were easy, everyone would be doing it! But guess what? YOU ARE DOING IT RIGHT NOW!

CHANGE YOUR ATTITUDE & PERSPECTIVE.

MEAL	TIME	WHAT DID YOU EAT? (INCLUDE ANY APPLICABLE SUPPLEMENTS)	NOTES*
BREAKFAST			
SNACK			
LUNCH			
SNACK			
DINNER			
SNACK			

*Examples: How do you feel? Did the food taste good or bad?
Was it a new recipe, preparation style, or spice? Any other comments.

HOW MUCH WATER DID I HAVE TODAY?
Remember: 128 ounces = 1 gallon = 16 cups = a well hydrated body

EXERCISE ACTIVITY	TIME SPENT	NOTES*

*Examples: How do you feel? Was an activity easy or challenging? Did you gain any strength or endurance?
Any other comments.

WRITE A DESCRIPTION OF YOUR FAVORITE POSITIVE MOMENT FROM TODAY:
Remember: It's up to you to create your positive environment and draw out your inner strength. Recognize any positivity surrounding you. Find it. Create it. Celebrate it. Daily.

SOMETIMES THE JOURNEY can be tough and old habits can sneak in without you realizing it. Take the weekend to work on food preparation, so you're prepared for the week. Also, do something physically fun: go on an exciting walk, take a trail hike, play basketball, go to the park, play with kids, go swimming or dancing, or practice yoga. Have fun, while still staying on your path.

BE GRATEFUL, EVERY DAY.

MEAL	TIME	WHAT DID YOU EAT? (INCLUDE ANY APPLICABLE SUPPLEMENTS)	NOTES*
BREAKFAST			
SNACK			
LUNCH			
SNACK			
DINNER			
SNACK			

*Examples: How do you feel? Did the food taste good or bad? Was it a new recipe, preparation style, or spice? Any other comments.

HOW MUCH WATER DID I HAVE TODAY?
Remember: 128 ounces = 1 gallon = 16 cups = a well hydrated body

EXERCISE ACTIVITY	TIME SPENT	NOTES*

*Examples: How do you feel? Was an activity easy or challenging? Did you gain any strength or endurance? Any other comments.

WRITE A DESCRIPTION OF YOUR FAVORITE POSITIVE MOMENT FROM TODAY:
Remember: It's up to you to create your positive environment and draw out your inner strength. Recognize any positivity surrounding you. Find it. Create it. Celebrate it. Daily.

Day 28/42

YOU CHOOSE YOUR PATH. You're gaining confidence and strength. Keep moving forward. Keep digging deeper, one step at a time. Record any of your Non-Scale Victories (p. XXX) and your body measurements (p. XXIX). If you choose, also take pictures of yourself to capture your transformation.

DON'T FORGET TO REST.

MEAL	TIME	WHAT DID YOU EAT? (INCLUDE ANY APPLICABLE SUPPLEMENTS)	NOTES*
BREAKFAST			
SNACK			
LUNCH			
SNACK			
DINNER			
SNACK			

*Examples: How do you feel? Did the food taste good or bad?
Was it a new recipe, preparation style, or spice? Any other comments.

HOW MUCH WATER DID I HAVE TODAY?
Remember: 128 ounces = 1 gallon = 16 cups = a well hydrated body

EXERCISE ACTIVITY	TIME SPENT	NOTES*

*Examples: How do you feel? Was an activity easy or challenging? Did you gain any strength or endurance?
Any other comments.

WRITE A DESCRIPTION OF YOUR FAVORITE POSITIVE MOMENT FROM TODAY:
Remember: It's up to you to create your positive environment and draw out your inner strength. Recognize any positivity surrounding you. Find it. Create it. Celebrate it. Daily.

I can **FEEL.**

I can **BE VULNERABLE.**

I can **HURT.**

I am **SAFE.**

I am **STRONG.**

I am **COMMITTED.**

I deserve **A HEALTHY BODY.**

I deserve **HAPPINESS.**

I deserve **PEACE.**

I am.

I am ***ME!***

Write your own affirmation:
(You can choose one from above or something new. Write anything that is meaningful and inspirational for you.)

WEEK 5: NO EXCUSES. WHAT'S STOPPING YOU?

"Do. Or do not. There is no try."
– **Jedi Master Yoda**

"Nothing can stop the man with the right mental attitude from achieving his goal; nothing on earth can help the man with the wrong mental attitude."
– **Thomas Jefferson**

You have come so far! Do you still have the motivation and drive to keep going? What can possibly stop you from getting to where you want to be? And what can you do about it? Make yourself—and your health-style—a priority. REFUSE TO GIVE UP. Week 5 can potentially be more difficult than the previous weeks for some. Your mind might want to play tricks on you. This could be a last-ditch effort of your old self, who wants to come out and play, to bring back your old, unhealthy habits. Why would you possibly want to go back there after all your efforts, sweat, and tears? Trust the process and keep moving forward!

Think of a time when you overcame a difficult challenge. Or think of a time when you performed your best work and felt proud. Or think of a time when you showed a positive attitude which made a difference for those around you, and perhaps lifted their spirits. Can you see that you have succeeded in the past in many different areas of your life? Apply this same mental strength, which you've proven you already have inside of you, to your health-style path.

Creating your new health-style really is mind over matter. The mind can try to tell your body to quit way too soon, when—if you really want to—you can go for a little longer in your workout; get in one more set or repetition; or stick to the nutrition plan when you really do not feel like it. A study on the development and maintenance of mental toughness conducted by the University of Wales Institute

115

found that pushing yourself to the limit, using long-term training goals as a source of motivation, and with a positive attitude, allowed new performers to strengthen their mental toughness.[1]

Can you think of any long-term training goals you want to reach? What is your attitude today? Building up tougher mind-over-matter abilities can also be achieved by establishing daily habits which allow you to be consistent with your goals in mind. Develop a clear system to help yourself stick with a schedule no matter how many excuses come up. Some examples of developing a schedule include: preparing your food on the same day each week, laying out your workout clothes and shoes before bed, attending the gym at the same time every day, and even setting the alarm and getting out of bed at the same time every day. Can you think of a few examples that work for you?

Experiencing any bumps in the road? Even Thomas Edison admitted: "I haven't failed. I've just found 10,000 ways that won't work." Skipping workouts, getting off track on your food plan, not giving 100% in the gym, or gaining a few pounds can just happen. Making mistakes is part of the process. Making mistakes is part of life. And this is how we learn and grow and become better at what we do. "Our greatest glory is not in never failing, but in RISING up every time we fail," said Ralph Waldo Emerson. We all experience challenges along the way and, yes, some are more severe than others. However, a bump is a bump. Simply walk over it and keep moving forward. Keep your attitude in check. You can recover from any setbacks or roadblocks in your path if you choose to.

Inspiration is an essential tool to successfully achieving your purpose. What inspires you? Inspiration will fuel the flames of your motivation.[2] This is important when you feel challenged or you are losing site of staying on track with your health-style path. Are you inspired by a photo or a favorite quote? If so, post it someplace where you can see it every day. I have photos posted on the refrigerator—as well as on the bathroom and bedroom mirrors! I also keep a folder on my computer of favorite quotes and constantly save them to my cell phone. Are you inspired by a particular person? Learn more about him or her. What are his or her drivers and motivating factors? Do you have sports role models? Read more about them, their teams, and their coaches. How do they train and eat—and why? What habits do they have to stay on path during times of stress or defeat? Are you inspired by any particular books? Read them! Go through your own journal entries in this very book and be inspired by your own journey. Look how far you have come. Look at what you have achieved. Look at what you are capable of. The important thing is to reignite your inspiration every day.

---

1   Declan Connaughton and Sheldon Hanton, et al, "The Development and Maintenance of Mental Toughness in the Word's Best Per-formers," *The Sport Psychologist* 24 (2010): 168-193.

2   Todd M. Thrash and Andrew J. Elliot, "Inspiration as a psychological construct," *Journal of Personality and Social Psychology* 84 (2003): 871-889.

Continue to educate yourself as you move through your journey. The more you know, the more power you will have. You will be inspired and motivated to stay the course by learning more specific details about clean eating, nutrition, and fitness. You have the world at your fingertips with modern technology. Explore blogs, websites, and support groups. Read fitness books, magazines, and journals. Join groups around town such as walking groups, running groups, or hiking groups. Go to a local sports store and check out the bulletin board to find any seminars, presentations, and talks that are happening around town. There is always something new to learn. Learn all that you can to feed your inspiration!

CAN'T STOP. WON'T EVER STOP.

List every excuse and reason you can think of for NOT making your health-style a priority in your life.

(For Mary's journal entry, see Appendix B)

_____

What actions can you take to get back on track when you start making excuses?

(For Mary's journal entry, see Appendix B)

_____

Imagine getting back on track after making excuses to quit. How would this make you feel?

(For Mary's journal entry, see Appendix B)

_____

Who or what can stop you from achieving your goals and adopting a new health-style for the long term? What are you going to do about it?

(For Mary's journal entry, see Appendix B)

_____

Real life adventures! What would you do?

Consider this scenario:

You lost twenty-six pounds during the first six weeks of your health-style journey. It is currently month three and you find yourself progressively getting busier with work and family responsibilities. You are only exercising twice a week and are slipping into old nutritional habits. You have gained ten pounds back. You ask yourself: "How did this happen?"

Why is getting back on track relevant to your life? How do you put yourself back on track? Do you struggle with motivation? What do you do about it? What triggers and behaviors do you need to be aware of?

THIS IS MONDAY, DAY 29. Let's double check the completion of your activities. Put a checkmark next to each item you've completed.

_____ **Logged a Daily Positive Moment for Week 4**

_____ **Logged a Daily Meal, Hydration, and Exercise Plan for Week 4**

_____ **Filled in your Body Measurments for Week 4** *p. XXIX*

_____ **Listed your Non-Scale Victories for Week 4** *p. XXX*

_____ **Filled in your Monday, Day 29, Weight** *p. XXXII*

_____ **Took applicable pictures for Week 4 (if you chose)**

_____ **Read "Week 5: No Excuses. What's Stopping You?"** *p. 115*

_____ **Answered the questions in "Can't Stop. Won't Ever Stop."** *p. 119*

_____ **Answered the questions in "What Would You Do?"** *p. 123*

DAILY LOG ENTRY
Day 29/42

THIS JOURNEY is about you and your own goals. You've come a long way, haven't you? Please do not compare your journey to any other journey out there. Your story is yours alone. Own it. Embrace it. Celebrate it. You are worth it. You got this. Never ever give up. Give it all you've got. Nothing can stop you.

DO IT FOR ME.

MEAL	TIME	WHAT DID YOU EAT? (INCLUDE ANY APPLICABLE SUPPLEMENTS)	NOTES*
BREAKFAST			
SNACK			
LUNCH			
SNACK			
DINNER			
SNACK			

*Examples: How do you feel? Did the food taste good or bad?
Was it a new recipe, preparation style, or spice? Any other comments.

HOW MUCH WATER DID I HAVE TODAY?
Remember: 128 ounces = 1 gallon = 16 cups = a well hydrated body

EXERCISE ACTIVITY	TIME SPENT	NOTES*

*Examples: How do you feel? Was an activity easy or challenging? Did you gain any strength or endurance?
Any other comments.

WRITE A DESCRIPTION OF YOUR FAVORITE POSITIVE MOMENT FROM TODAY:
Remember: It's up to you to create your positive environment and draw out your inner strength. Recognize any positivity surrounding you. Find it. Create it. Celebrate it. Daily.

DAILY LOG ENTRY

EVERY SUCCESS is fueled by mind over matter. Surround yourself with truth, accountability, support, trust, and empowerment. What do those mean for you? Keep up the positive momentum in your journey. Stay engaged with gym buddies or any friends and/or family who positively support your path.

MOVE PAST THE PAIN.

MEAL	TIME	WHAT DID YOU EAT? (INCLUDE ANY APPLICABLE SUPPLEMENTS)	NOTES*
BREAKFAST			
SNACK			
LUNCH			
SNACK			
DINNER			
SNACK			

*Examples: How do you feel? Did the food taste good or bad?
Was it a new recipe, preparation style, or spice? Any other comments.

HOW MUCH WATER DID I HAVE TODAY?
Remember: 128 ounces = 1 gallon = 16 cups = a well hydrated body

EXERCISE ACTIVITY	TIME SPENT	NOTES*

*Examples: How do you feel? Was an activity easy or challenging? Did you gain any strength or endurance?
Any other comments.

WRITE A DESCRIPTION OF YOUR FAVORITE POSITIVE MOMENT FROM TODAY:
Remember: It's up to you to create your positive environment and draw out your inner strength. Recognize any positivity surrounding you. Find it. Create it. Celebrate it. Daily.

CONTINUE TO LEARN. The more you know, the more power you will have. Educate yourself on clean eating and nutrition. Understand how to continue this lifestyle for the long term. Learn about the human body, kinesiology, or various forms of exercise. Read online and get books and magazines. Learn all you can!

GROW CONFIDENCE AND SELF-ESTEEM.

MEAL	TIME	WHAT DID YOU EAT? (INCLUDE ANY APPLICABLE SUPPLEMENTS)	NOTES*
BREAKFAST			
SNACK			
LUNCH			
SNACK			
DINNER			
SNACK			

*Examples: How do you feel? Did the food taste good or bad?
Was it a new recipe, preparation style, or spice? Any other comments.

HOW MUCH WATER DID I HAVE TODAY?
Remember: 128 ounces = 1 gallon = 16 cups = a well hydrated body

EXERCISE ACTIVITY	TIME SPENT	NOTES*

*Examples: How do you feel? Was an activity easy or challenging? Did you gain any strength or endurance? Any other comments.

WRITE A DESCRIPTION OF YOUR FAVORITE POSITIVE MOMENT FROM TODAY:
Remember: It's up to you to create your positive environment and draw out your inner strength. Recognize any positivity surrounding you. Find it. Create it. Celebrate it. Daily.

Day 32/42

CONTINUE TO SET MINI-GOALS for yourself.

These will keep you motivated to keep moving forward. Once you reach a goal, celebrate it—and then set another one. Specific and measureable mini-goals will keep you accountable when you can achieve them in a timely manner. Give yourself more to celebrate along the way!

COMMITMENT, DEDICATION & PERSISTENCE!

MEAL	TIME	WHAT DID YOU EAT? (INCLUDE ANY APPLICABLE SUPPLEMENTS)	NOTES*
BREAKFAST			
SNACK			
LUNCH			
SNACK			
DINNER			
SNACK			

*Examples: How do you feel? Did the food taste good or bad?
Was it a new recipe, preparation style, or spice? Any other comments.

HOW MUCH WATER DID I HAVE TODAY?
Remember: 128 ounces = 1 gallon = 16 cups = a well hydrated body

EXERCISE ACTIVITY	TIME SPENT	NOTES*

*Examples: How do you feel? Was an activity easy or challenging? Did you gain any strength or endurance?
Any other comments.

WRITE A DESCRIPTION OF YOUR FAVORITE POSITIVE MOMENT FROM TODAY:
Remember: It's up to you to create your positive environment and draw out your inner strength. Recognize any positivity surrounding you. Find it. Create it. Celebrate it. Daily.

Day 33/42

REIGNITE YOUR INSPIRATION every day.

What inspires you? Is it your child, spouse, family, or religion? Are you inspired by reading the paper, a good novel, or a religious book? Does inspiration come from meditation or taking a few minutes to yourself? Whatever connects you with inspiration, carve out some time to keep it fresh in your mind!

HARD WORK PAYS OFF!

MEAL	TIME	WHAT DID YOU EAT? (INCLUDE ANY APPLICABLE SUPPLEMENTS)	NOTES*
BREAKFAST			
SNACK			
LUNCH			
SNACK			
DINNER			
SNACK			

*Examples: How do you feel? Did the food taste good or bad?
Was it a new recipe, preparation style, or spice? Any other comments.

HOW MUCH WATER DID I HAVE TODAY?
Remember: 128 ounces = 1 gallon = 16 cups = a well hydrated body

EXERCISE ACTIVITY	TIME SPENT	NOTES*

*Examples: How do you feel? Was an activity easy or challenging? Did you gain any strength or endurance?
Any other comments.

WRITE A DESCRIPTION OF YOUR FAVORITE POSITIVE MOMENT FROM TODAY:
Remember: It's up to you to create your positive environment and draw out your inner strength. Recognize any positivity surrounding you. Find it. Create it. Celebrate it. Daily.

THE WEEKEND is here! What are you going to do with it to prepare you for the final week of your six-week journey? Are you ready to give it all you've got? Do not sabotage yourself this weekend. You have come too far to slip into old habits now. Review your journal entries throughout this book and consider what an incredible journey you've had. Keep the party going!

YOUR ACCOUNTABILITY PAYS OFF!

MEAL	TIME	WHAT DID YOU EAT? (INCLUDE ANY APPLICABLE SUPPLEMENTS)	NOTES*
BREAKFAST			
SNACK			
LUNCH			
SNACK			
DINNER			
SNACK			

*Examples: How do you feel? Did the food taste good or bad?
Was it a new recipe, preparation style, or spice? Any other comments.

HOW MUCH WATER DID I HAVE TODAY?
Remember: 128 ounces = 1 gallon = 16 cups = a well hydrated body

EXERCISE ACTIVITY	TIME SPENT	NOTES*

*Examples: How do you feel? Was an activity easy or challenging? Did you gain any strength or endurance?
Any other comments.

WRITE A DESCRIPTION OF YOUR FAVORITE POSITIVE MOMENT FROM TODAY:
Remember: It's up to you to create your positive environment and draw out your inner strength. Recognize any positivity surrounding you. Find it. Create it. Celebrate it. Daily.

Day 35 / 42

FOOD PREPARATION Today is the day to celebrate any new Non-Scale Victories (p. XXX) and your body measurements (p. XXIX). Have you formed a habit of celebrating end-of-the-week victories? What other daily and weekly habits have been helping you along the way? If you choose, remember to take pictures of yourself today. [See Appendix A for some healthy celebration ideas.]

YOU ARE WORTH IT!

MEAL	TIME	WHAT DID YOU EAT? (INCLUDE ANY APPLICABLE SUPPLEMENTS)	NOTES*
BREAKFAST			
SNACK			
LUNCH			
SNACK			
DINNER			
SNACK			

*Examples: How do you feel? Did the food taste good or bad?
Was it a new recipe, preparation style, or spice? Any other comments.

HOW MUCH WATER DID I HAVE TODAY?
Remember: 128 ounces = 1 gallon = 16 cups = a well hydrated body

EXERCISE ACTIVITY	TIME SPENT	NOTES*

*Examples: How do you feel? Was an activity easy or challenging? Did you gain any strength or endurance?
Any other comments.

WRITE A DESCRIPTION OF YOUR FAVORITE POSITIVE MOMENT FROM TODAY:
Remember: It's up to you to create your positive environment and draw out your inner strength. Recognize any positivity surrounding you. Find it. Create it. Celebrate it. Daily.

No **EXCUSES.**

No **DRAMA.**

No **DARKNESS.**

Yes, **THERE WILL BE CHALLENGES.**

Yes, **THERE WILL BE STRUGGLE.**

Yes, **THERE WILL BE CRAVINGS FOR OLD HABITS.**

My past **DOES NOT DEFINE MY FUTURE.**

I choose **MY PATH.**

I will **OVERCOME.**

I will **LIVE A HEALTHY LIFE.**

I can **DO THIS!**

Write your own affirmation:
(You can choose one from above or something new. Write anything that is meaningful and inspirational for you.)

WEEK 6: DESIGNING YOUR FUTURE—WHAT'S NEXT?

"There is a difference between interest and commitment. When you're interested in doing something, you do it only when it's convenient. When you're committed to something, you accept no excuses, only results."
– **Kenneth H. Blanchard**

"The best way to predict the future is to create it."
– **Abraham Lincoln**

How many people have the courage to change their lives for the better? I do not know, but you are one of them! It is time to start envisioning your future. Where do you want to be three weeks, three months, six months, or even a year from now? What does that health-style look like? What does it feel like? Do these images bring a smile to your face? What tools do you need to reach your goals? Do you need a gym membership as a tool? Do you need more recipe books or cooking classes to support and broaden your healthy eating? Are you starting to think about future mini-goals to get you to where you want to be?

Your work in this journal has built up inner strength and momentum for you to keep going and smash it to the end. What does it take to build up momentum? It takes: understanding your "why?"; learning about food, nutrition, and exercise; knowing what you want and the benefits your goals bring you; being empowered with habits and tools to combat any excuses that stand in your way; and keeping a positive attitude and going for it. This 6-week, 42-day journey is a jumpstart to your new beginning . . . to your new chapter . . . to your new *life*. Who doesn't want to be healthy, happy, energetic, and strong?

Whether in fitness, career, health, school, or other areas of your life, setting goals creates a cycle of success, which leads to increased efforts, higher self-esteem, more involvement, and setting even more goals to drive you forward.[1] How does one go about developing and setting goals in general? The acronym SMART is a common method used today in managerial goal setting. The letters in SMART refer to: Specific, Measurable, Achievable, Relevant, and Timely.[2] As applied to health and fitness, the SMART goals in more detail need to be:

Specific. What exactly do you want to accomplish? *(Lose weight)* How much weight? *(Ten pounds)* Why do you want to set this goal? *(To be in a healthy body mass index range)* What are the resources needed? *(Gym access and clean-eating foods)*

Measureable. Every goal needs to be quantifiable for specific tracking. For example, weight loss can be measured on a scale, fat loss or muscle gains can use a combination of weight tracking along with body measurements and/or fat caliper measurements.

Achievable. Is the goal realistic? Will it challenge you? Are there any constraints to consider? For example, imagine that you have set the endurance goal to be able to row on a rowing machine for one hour without stopping. However, you have no access (gym or otherwise) to a rowing machine. This would not be an *achievable* goal due to lack of resources.

Relevant. Does the specific goal matter (or seem worthwhile) to you? For example, imagine that your true intent is to increase muscle mass. It would not be relevant to set a goal of running an eight-minute mile. Is your specific goal relevant to your overall desires?

Timely. Can you achieve your goal in a realistic timeframe? For example, setting a goal to lose twenty pounds in ten days is not realistic for most.

With a different perspective, another fun acronym, "SWOT," will also get you thinking about your specific health and fitness goals. SWOT stands for: Strengths, Weaknesses, Opportunities, and Threats. If that sounds familiar, it's because you have already done permutations of both SMART goal setting and SWOT analysis throughout this guide! SWOT analysis is adapted here to be used toward your health-style path. Consider the following when planning your health and fitness goals:

---

1   Douglas T. Hall and Lawrence W. Foster, "A Psychological Success Cycle and Goal Setting: Goals, Performance, and Attitudes," *Academy of Management Journal* 20, no. 2 (1977): pages 282-290.

2   George T. Doran, "There's a S.M.A.R.T. way to write management's goals and objectives," *Management Review* 70, no. 11 (1981): pages 35-36.

Strengths. What are your personal strengths to accomplish the specific health-style goal?

Weaknesses. What are your personal challenges and obstacles? Are there any roadblocks that can stand in your way? What do you have to be on the lookout for as you work on your goal? What can you do about it?

Opportunities. What are the benefits of your goal? What will they get you? Are there any ways to exploit and maximize these benefits? How can you strengthen and build upon these benefits?

Threats. Are there any external factors that stand in the way of achieving your goal (such as a negative environment, lack of support, lack of access to a gym or home program, a bad work schedule, family responsibilities, etc.)? What can you do about them?

Remember to have fun in the process of setting, working toward, and achieving your goals. This is your health-style path. There is something to be said about stopping and smelling the roses! This is a journey. This is a life-style change. Enjoy it. Embrace it. Live it. Above all, get out there and *do* it!

MAKING IT A LIFESTYLE.

What strengths have you uncovered within you?
(For Mary's journal entry, see Appendix B)

List your top favorite "wins" since starting this new path (goals achieved, scale and/or Non-Scale Victories, etc.). Why are these significant to you?

(For Mary's journal entry, see Appendix B)

_____

List your top learnings/insights realized on this journey so far. Can these insights help you further? How?

(For Mary's journal entry, see Appendix B)

_____

How will you continue your nutritional and exercise goals moving forward? Will you start/continue with a gym membership or exercise program? How will you integrate a healthy eating style for the long term? List your planned actions.

(For Mary's journal entry, see Appendix B)

_____

Where do you want to be in your health and fitness journey, three weeks from now? Three months from now? Six months from now? One year from now?

(For Mary's journal entry, see Appendix B)

_____

Three weeks:

Three months:

Six months:

One year:

You have one more week to go on your current six-week journey. How are you feeling? Do you have any concerns, fears, or demotivating factors? If so, list them here. Ask yourself "Why do these exist?" Now write any actions you can take to counteract them.

(For Mary's journal entry, see Appendix B)

_____

THIS IS MONDAY, DAY 36. Let's double check the completion of your activities. Put a checkmark next to each item you've completed.

_____ **Logged a Daily Positive Moment for Week 5**

_____ **Logged a Daily Meal, Hydration, and Exercise Plan for Week 5**

_____ **Filled in your Body Measurments for Week 5** *p. XXIX*

_____ **Listed your Non-Scale Victories for Week 5** *p. XXX*

_____ **Filled in your Monday, Day 36, Weight** *p. XXXII*

_____ **Took applicable pictures for Week 5 (if you chose)**

_____ **Read "Week 6: Designing Your Future—Whats Next?"** *p. 143*

_____ **Answered the questions in "Making It a Lifestyle"** *p. 147*

Day 36/42

WHAT DO YOU WANT? How do you want to live your life? How do you envision your health-style three years from now? What are the benefits to all of this? Why are you on this path? Why continue this path? What is stopping you? Seriously, what do you really want? Now go out there and get it. It can be yours!

DO YOUR ULTIMATE BEST.

MEAL	TIME	WHAT DID YOU EAT? (INCLUDE ANY APPLICABLE SUPPLEMENTS)	NOTES*
BREAKFAST			
SNACK			
LUNCH			
SNACK			
DINNER			
SNACK			

*Examples: How do you feel? Did the food taste good or bad?
Was it a new recipe, preparation style, or spice? Any other comments.

HOW MUCH WATER DID I HAVE TODAY?
Remember: 128 ounces = 1 gallon = 16 cups = a well hydrated body

EXERCISE ACTIVITY	TIME SPENT	NOTES*

*Examples: How do you feel? Was an activity easy or challenging? Did you gain any strength or endurance? Any other comments.

WRITE A DESCRIPTION OF YOUR FAVORITE POSITIVE MOMENT FROM TODAY:
Remember: It's up to you to create your positive environment and draw out your inner strength. Recognize any positivity surrounding you. Find it. Create it. Celebrate it. Daily.

Day 37/42

WHAT IS A ROADBLOCK, but a bump in the road? Challenges, obstacles, and old habits can come up and get us off track. You have the power, knowledge, strength, and mental will to get back up, get on track, and overcome any roadblock that is thrown your way. You have proven that this health-style is achievable.

REACH OUT FOR HELP.

MEAL	TIME	WHAT DID YOU EAT? (INCLUDE ANY APPLICABLE SUPPLEMENTS)	NOTES*
BREAKFAST			
SNACK			
LUNCH			
SNACK			
DINNER			
SNACK			

*Examples: How do you feel? Did the food taste good or bad?
Was it a new recipe, preparation style, or spice? Any other comments.

HOW MUCH WATER DID I HAVE TODAY?
Remember: 128 ounces = 1 gallon = 16 cups = a well hydrated body

EXERCISE ACTIVITY	TIME SPENT	NOTES*

*Examples: How do you feel? Was an activity easy or challenging? Did you gain any strength or endurance? Any other comments.

WRITE A DESCRIPTION OF YOUR FAVORITE POSITIVE MOMENT FROM TODAY:
Remember: It's up to you to create your positive environment and draw out your inner strength. Recognize any positivity surrounding you. Find it. Create it. Celebrate it. Daily.

GET CREATIVE in the various ways you can hold yourself accountable to your goals. Do stress or emotions influence your choices? How can you stay accountable for your health-style during these times? This can now be a long-term lifestyle if you want it to be. No excuses. What is stopping you?

NO OPTION OF QUITTING.

MEAL	TIME	WHAT DID YOU EAT? (INCLUDE ANY APPLICABLE SUPPLEMENTS)	NOTES*
BREAKFAST			
SNACK			
LUNCH			
SNACK			
DINNER			
SNACK			

*Examples: How do you feel? Did the food taste good or bad?
Was it a new recipe, preparation style, or spice? Any other comments.

HOW MUCH WATER DID I HAVE TODAY?
Remember: 128 ounces = 1 gallon = 16 cups = a well hydrated body

EXERCISE ACTIVITY	TIME SPENT	NOTES*

*Examples: How do you feel? Was an activity easy or challenging? Did you gain any strength or endurance? Any other comments.

WRITE A DESCRIPTION OF YOUR FAVORITE POSITIVE MOMENT FROM TODAY:
Remember: It's up to you to create your positive environment and draw out your inner strength. Recognize any positivity surrounding you. Find it. Create it. Celebrate it. Daily.

REMEMBER TO HAVE FUN when setting, working toward, and achieving your goals. Have you found an exercise or activity that you like doing? Do more of that! Can you recruit friends or family to share in the fun? Have you found a new favorite spice? Or a new favorite clean meal? Keep exploring that. Enjoy—and be happy!

DO NOT LOSE FAITH!

MEAL	TIME	WHAT DID YOU EAT? (INCLUDE ANY APPLICABLE SUPPLEMENTS)	NOTES*
BREAKFAST			
SNACK			
LUNCH			
SNACK			
DINNER			
SNACK			

*Examples: How do you feel? Did the food taste good or bad?
Was it a new recipe, preparation style, or spice? Any other comments.

HOW MUCH WATER DID I HAVE TODAY?
Remember: 128 ounces = 1 gallon = 16 cups = a well hydrated body

EXERCISE ACTIVITY	TIME SPENT	NOTES*

*Examples: How do you feel? Was an activity easy or challenging? Did you gain any strength or endurance?
Any other comments.

WRITE A DESCRIPTION OF YOUR FAVORITE POSITIVE MOMENT FROM TODAY:
Remember: It's up to you to create your positive environment and draw out your inner strength. Recognize any positivity surrounding you. Find it. Create it. Celebrate it. Daily.

GIVE SOME BACK.

You have almost completed six weeks of a new, healthy lifestyle. You have lived, learned, and conquered many victories along the way. Share your learnings with friends and family. Inspire those around you. Encourage health and well-being in your world. Fill the air with a healthy attitude!

IT'S ALL IN THE ATTITUDE!

MEAL	TIME	WHAT DID YOU EAT? (INCLUDE ANY APPLICABLE SUPPLEMENTS)	NOTES*
BREAKFAST			
SNACK			
LUNCH			
SNACK			
DINNER			
SNACK			

*Examples: How do you feel? Did the food taste good or bad?
Was it a new recipe, preparation style, or spice? Any other comments.

HOW MUCH WATER DID I HAVE TODAY?
Remember: 128 ounces = 1 gallon = 16 cups = a well hydrated body

EXERCISE ACTIVITY	TIME SPENT	NOTES*

*Examples: How do you feel? Was an activity easy or challenging? Did you gain any strength or endurance?
Any other comments.

WRITE A DESCRIPTION OF YOUR FAVORITE POSITIVE MOMENT FROM TODAY:
Remember: It's up to you to create your positive environment and draw out your inner strength. Recognize any positivity surrounding you. Find it. Create it. Celebrate it. Daily.

DAILY LOG ENTRY

GOT HEALTH-STYLE? Look how far you have come. Embrace and enjoy the weekend. Have fun with it. You know how to eat clean. Got Health-Style? You know how to set goals and stick with an exercise plan. You have done this. You are doing this. Got Health-Style? Yes, of course you do!

ALWAYS *ALWAYS* FOLLOW THROUGH.

MEAL	TIME	WHAT DID YOU EAT? (INCLUDE ANY APPLICABLE SUPPLEMENTS)	NOTES*
BREAKFAST			
SNACK			
LUNCH			
SNACK			
DINNER			
SNACK			

*Examples: How do you feel? Did the food taste good or bad?
Was it a new recipe, preparation style, or spice? Any other comments.

HOW MUCH WATER DID I HAVE TODAY?
Remember: 128 ounces = 1 gallon = 16 cups = a well hydrated body

EXERCISE ACTIVITY	TIME SPENT	NOTES*

*Examples: How do you feel? Was an activity easy or challenging? Did you gain any strength or endurance?
Any other comments.

WRITE A DESCRIPTION OF YOUR FAVORITE POSITIVE MOMENT FROM TODAY:
Remember: It's up to you to create your positive environment and draw out your inner strength. Recognize any positivity surrounding you. Find it. Create it. Celebrate it. Daily.

YAHOO! YOU MADE IT!

You did it! You conquered it! Well done! If you want, this can be the beginning of your great new life. Honor any Non-Scale Victories this week (p. XXX) and record your body measurements (p. XXIX). Surely take pictures of yourself today to celebrate. Praise all of the dedication and commitment that got you here. Congratulations!

IT CAN BE DONE!

MEAL	TIME	WHAT DID YOU EAT? (INCLUDE ANY APPLICABLE SUPPLEMENTS)	NOTES*
BREAKFAST			
SNACK			
LUNCH			
SNACK			
DINNER			
SNACK			

*Examples: How do you feel? Did the food taste good or bad?
Was it a new recipe, preparation style, or spice? Any other comments.

HOW MUCH WATER DID I HAVE TODAY?
Remember: 128 ounces = 1 gallon = 16 cups = a well hydrated body

EXERCISE ACTIVITY	TIME SPENT	NOTES*

*Examples: How do you feel? Was an activity easy or challenging? Did you gain any strength or endurance?
Any other comments.

WRITE A DESCRIPTION OF YOUR FAVORITE POSITIVE MOMENT FROM TODAY:
Remember: It's up to you to create your positive environment and draw out your inner strength. Recognize any positivity surrounding you. Find it. Create it. Celebrate it. Daily.

THIS IS MONDAY, DAY 43. WE MADE IT TO THE END!!! Let's double check the completion of your activities. Put a checkmark next to each item you've completed.

_____ **Logged a Daily Positive Moment for Week 6**

_____ **Logged a Daily Meal, Hydration, and Exercise Plan for Week 6**

_____ **Filled in your Body Measurments for Week 6** *p. XXIX*

_____ **Listed your Non-Scale Victories for Week 6** *p. XXX*

_____ **Filled in your Monday, Day 43, END WEIGHT** *p. XXXII*

_____ **Took applicable pictures for Week 6 (if you chose)**

_____ **Read "Conclusions"** *p. 173*

_____ **Log your entries in "My Journey is only beginning"** *p. 176*

_____ **Write your affirmations to "Inspire Yourself Forward"** *p. 175*

I choose **MY HEALTH-STYLE PATH.**

I choose **TO BE AWARE OF THE PRESENT.**

I choose **TO LIVE NOW.**

I will **BE CHALLENGED.**

I will **OVERCOME.**

I will **BE TEMPTED.**

I will **PERSERVERE.**

No excuses **CAN HOLD ME BACK.**

No roadblock **WILL STOP ME.**

I am me. **I AM ME. I AM ME!**

I am ***DOING THIS!***

Write your own affirmation:
(You can choose one from above or something new. Write anything that is
meaningful and inspirational for you.)

CONCLUSIONS

"Success is not final, failure is not fatal: it is the courage to continue that counts."
– **Winston Churchill**

Congratulations! You have completed your six-week jumpstart to embracing a new, healthy lifestyle. You made it. You did it. You committed, saw it through over the finish line, and are now at the starting line to your future. What does health-style mean for you as you think about the future? What do you want? (No, really.) What do you *really* want as you continue moving forward? How will that benefit you? What do you get out of it? How important is this lifestyle to you? What is stopping you from getting there? Anything is possible. Did you ever dream of running a half marathon, taking up a physical hobby, jumping out of an airplane, wearing a particular outfit, climbing a mountain, having a particular physique, or lifting a certain weight? Go out there and continue to go for it! Dream—and then make it happen.

Do you feel closer to your inner power? What can you do to get further connected to it? By what means are you going to apply your strengths toward the future? Do you feel more comfortable and responsible for conquering personal challenges and/or any roadblocks that could stand in your way? What will you do about them? Will you continue to hold yourself accountable for your nutrition and exercise plan as well as accountable for mini- and long-term goals? If yes, by what means will you hold yourself accountable? If no, why the heck not? Will you continue to foster a positive attitude and build a positive environment around you? You made it for six weeks, so why quit now?

"Health. Family. Job. This is the order of priorities to live by." This is advice from Richard B., a former boss and mentor of mine—from more than six years ago. I did not fully understand what was being said back then. It took me going through severe health battles with cancer and lupus—along with my own health-style struggles—to understand the power of that statement. It now resonates within me. What do those priorities mean for you?

Another nugget shared with me by Richard (who acquired this advice from his own mentor thirty-plus years prior) is the acronym TASTE, which he used in corporate development-related tasks. TASTE in the context of our health-style journey is interpreted as the following:

Trust. Trust the process. Learn from mistakes. Mistakes and bumps in the road where you go off the path *happen*. For example, you may stop following your nutrition and exercise programs or gain a few pounds. What can you learn when mistakes and bumps occur?

Accountability. You have to come in with a plan, ready and prepared. Take ownership of your goals, attitude, and how you combat any obstacles. How will you hold yourself accountable?

Support. Support yourself. Be kind to yourself. Recognize all forms of victory, including Non-Scale Victories. Celebrate the wins.

Truth. Be truthful to yourself. Don't allow yourself to use any excuses. Only you really know if you are giving it your all. Can you look at yourself in the mirror and say that you are being truthful in pursuit of your health-style?

Empowerment. Use your strengths, talent, and motivational factors to make change happen and contribute to your positive environment.

TASTE your future. TASTE your life. TASTE your environment. TASTE your goals!

As you move forward, now it's time to consider what you can do for others. Can you inspire and empower others toward a health-style path as well? By what means can you contribute and give back, should you have the desire? Why not share and spread the positive, healthy lifestyle?

You deserve to be healthy. You deserve to be happy. You deserve to be strong. You deserve to be full of life energy. You deserve to be connected with your inner strength. Own your health-style path. Embrace your health-style. Be empowered. Empower others. Release your inner roar. Don't ever stop. Don't ever quit. You can do this!

INSPIRE YOURSELF FORWARD.

Write your affirmations from previous pages here.
Use your own words to motivate and inspire yourself
to continue your long-term health-style path.

Page XXI:
_____

Page XXXIII:
_____

Page XLIII:
_____

Page LI:
_____

Page 27:
_____

Page 55:
_____

Page 85:
_____

Page 113:
_____

Page 141.
_____

Page 171:
_____

MY JOURNEY IS ONLY BEGINNING.

May love and joy fill your heart as you continue to live your new health-style. You possess the inner power and strength to achieve any goal. Release your beast and inner roar! I wish you sincere peace in mind, body, and soul.

Before you go, take a moment to reflect on this six-week journey and the beginnings of living your new health-style path. Use this page and the next to capture any thoughts, feelings, and important lessons you have learned.

(For Mary's journal entry, see Appendix C)

NOTES

NOTES

NOTES

NOTES

APPENDIX A:
HEALTHY WAYS TO CELEBRATE

What are some healthy ways to celebrate? For many, celebrating means being rewarded with fatty and sugary foods, along with wine, beer, or other alcoholic drinks. While you can certainly enjoy these foods and drinks in moderation, there is no reason to use these items as a reward system. We need to find other ways to celebrate in a health-wise manner. After all, why should we celebrate and reward our health with something unhealthy?

Here are some alternative suggestions:

- Buy a new outfit
- Buy new exercise clothes
- Buy new running/workout shoes
- Buy ten new workout songs on iTunes
- Go dancing
- Get a babysitter and have date night with your significant other
- Have sex!
- Buy new (non-workout!) shoes or a new purse
- Get a manicure or pedicure
- Get a massage
- Get your hair done
- Enjoy a golf game, tennis game, or basketball game
- Get together with friends
- Go for a hike or on a camping trip
- Complete a home project you have always wanted to do
- Take time off to see a movie
- Take time off to read a book
- Take time to do your favorite hobby
- Take a long bubble bath
- Buy a new sports "toy" (new weight, tennis racket, soccer ball, etc.)
- Go play at the beach
- Plan a weekend getaway
- Plan a vacation

APPENDIX B: MARY'S JOURNAL ENTRIES

BEFORE DAY 1: WHAT IS YOUR "WHY"?

What do you want to accomplish in the next six weeks?

I want to lose twenty pounds and be more comfortable with my eating habits. I've been eating somewhat "healthy," but I don't feel like I know how to eat the right portions. I don't always feel in control of my eating and often crave sugary foods. I know I can overeat and give in to junk food pretty easily. Maybe I don't eat too healthy after all? I don't know.

I want to be able to get strong so that I feel "normal." My body is weak from all the months of bedrest these last two years, going thru 6 cancer-related surgeries, even after all the rehabbing. I still can't even lift my legs off the floor right now, even though I can walk miles! Guess it takes different muscles to lift up. six months ago, I was just learning to walk again and put on my own shoes.

I'm hoping to do something about my energy. I am sick and tired of being sick and tired all the time. Hopefully, this weight loss and more will help.

Why do you want a new health-style?

Something has to change. I have been overweight and yo-yoed up and down the scale since I was about ten years old. I'm sick of it. Never been able to keep any sort of weight off for more than two months! I gain it all back again and then some. I feel like I've tried every crazy diet possible. I am tired of feeling like a failure with this. I want to be strong. I want to look fit. I want to feel sexy! I've never felt pretty. I've always had a marshmallow body, and I have never had a single visible muscle on me!

I want a healthy and active life. I want to live a long life for my son and husband. I stay home on the couch when they go play at the park because I don't have enough energy to join in. I want to be part of the fun activities.

I've been given another chance to start my life anew after all the health drama these last 2 years. I don't want lupus to beat me, or have cancer come back. It's hard being active with rheumatoid arthritis, osteoarthritis, and colitis from lupus. When it flares, my guts, joints, and bones hurt.

My mom died at my age from complications of progressive multiple sclerosis (also an autoimmune disease). She was a full quadriplegic at the end. When I was a teenager, I watched her go from a cane, to a walker, to a wheelchair in just one year. She didn't even try to exercise or fight back. I don't want to be like that—not fighting back or trying.

What has stopped you before (what were your previous roadblocks)?

I usually end up quitting exercise programs. Go "all or nothing," pull a muscle or get hurt in some way, rest up to get better, and then never start again. Or get bored and make excuses to not do it. Or let general pain and health get in the way and not even try. It seems easier to just be tired.

I get busy with work and life and have no time. Well, I don't *make* the time. . . . Or I don't consciously think about my own needs, because I take care of everyone else's—my clients, my family, etc. I'm usually too busy working on some work goal, it seems. Then I'm just too tired to take care of me.

The diets that I have been on before were short-term solutions, and I didn't know what to do afterwards. I feel lost and don't exactly know how to approach a long-term eating style. I end up craving sweets and give in. When I get tired, I shove food in my face without thinking, whether I am hungry or not.

Even though I have food limitations and need to eat gluten free, soy free, and dairy free to manage the lupus inflammatory issues, I still manage to overload on not-so-healthy foods when I'm tired and stressed. Obviously, my *real* health issues of the last 2 years have stopped me too.

How will you overcome your roadblock(s) in the next six weeks?

I got a jumpstart fighting roadblocks from all the rehab. Many months to learn how to walk and move my arms and other body parts again, etc. It has been a lot of hard work to go from bedrest and not being able to stand, to walking 10 miles down the street! I lost about 40 pounds during the last 6 months as a result, probably due to the consistent rehab exercise and eating more healthy to increase my energy and general health.

I need to hold myself accountable and see this through to the end, so I signed up for a weight loss six-week challenge at my gym, The Camp Transformation Center. I hit a plateau 2 months ago, and normally would have given up by now. I've never met my ultimate weight goal before. I end up quitting and gain weight back. This time, I am hoping to learn more about clean eating so I can integrate it into my life for the long haul and make long-term life changes with guidance. Also, as part of my obligation to the gym challenge, I must work out 30 times in 42 days. Thus, I can't make any excuses to not stick with it.

What strengths do you have, which will enable you to reach your goal? (One way to consider this question is to imagine a previous success in any aspect of your life and draw upon what worked to make it successful.)

I had a tough childhood and made it through with determination and resilience. I was determined at a young age to not let circumstances mentally beat me down. One thing I give myself credit for is making it through the rabbit hole as well as I have!

In my professional and academic life as an adult, I am known for persistence, hard work, and never giving up. I was the first one in my immediate family to go to college (my mother didn't graduate high school). I even made it to graduate school and graduated with a doctorate.

Six years later, I decided to go to graduate school again for an executive MBA and managed to do pretty well, while being the first woman to have a baby in the middle of the program! There's nothing like an emergency C-section for delivery after 36 hours of labor and then going back to class for 12 hours/day less than two weeks later only to ace a Global Strategy exam! I'm proud of myself for pulling that off and for graduating on time with the rest of my class, while juggling a newborn baby! (Well, not literally!)

I've always been pretty determined if I set my mind to it and find this as my core strength. However, I never really took this attitude and energy to apply it directly to my own self-needs and health. It seems kinda weird when I really think about it. It always seemed like I had an *outward* determination to get things done—gain degrees, gain career titles, etc. But then, these last few years I was forced to draw on this energy and mindset to simply stay alive and to not let health issues beat me.

Until I almost died, I never really paid much attention to myself inwardly. I am a survivor. For the first time in my life, I am making the choice to put my health and fitness first, because *I want to*. Not because I have to in order to fight to stay alive. I am not going to let "IT" (whatever "IT" is) beat me! I will survive. And I will do this! I know I can do this. I have to. I really just have to get my body healthy and my mind right to keep it healthy. I have to do this, this time!

WEEK 1: WHAT IS YOUR RELATIONSHIP WITH NUTRITION?

What factors influenced your food choices before starting this six-week journey? Do stress or emotions typically influence your choices? Describe them and how they do so.

I have food limitations, as certain foods cause me severe inflammatory issues (this list includes soy, dairy, gluten, oats, buckwheat, apples, grapes, broccoli, kale, chicken, and some others). I like to cook and explore new spices. It is fun to go out and try new dishes and flavors, then attempt to reproduce them at home.

I love carbs: gluten-free pasta, bread, and sweet things. My husband is a vegetarian who eats fish. My son eats meat, but I don't cook it very often. Cane sugar gives me issues, so I try to use honey and maple syrup and other sweets instead. I seem to go through the "honey bear" pretty quickly.

I am surely an emotional eater! When I get sad, tired, or stressed I usually eat without realizing it. I go for sweet or fattening foods in this case. Sometimes, I'll just crave salty foods so I'll start to eat chips—and lots of them. I'll often snack mindlessly in front of the TV on movie nights. I will also reward myself with sweets.

And my food choices can be controlled by social functions. I generally eat a lot more than I need to at restaurants or get-togethers with friends or family.

What are the biggest nutritional challenges for you and your family?

Designing a meal that my family can all eat together is a challenge. I often cook extra side items for myself (such as making myself gluten-free pasta and the family regular pasta).

As a family, we don't seem to eat a lot of protein. This is partly because the hubby only eats fish as an animal protein and partly because I don't have much experience cooking meat—and I get a bit grossed out by handling raw meat. We also use beans, nuts, and dairy as a family protein source, but I have no idea how much we really get.

As a family, we collectively eat a lot of carbs right now. We eat lots of vegetables and fruit though. We like shopping at the local farmers' markets. I like to serve a colorful plate for dinner. Luckily, my son is not a picky eater and will generally eat what is set in front of him.

Have you ever considered the nutritional value of food when making food choices? Why or why not?

No, never thought about it. I can't eat a lot of prepared foods because of my limitations, so luckily a lot of junk food and processed food is automatically dismissed.

Besides looking at ingredient list to see if an item is on my "inflammatory list," I have never paid attention to how much protein, fat, or carbs a food item has in it. I really have NO IDEA about this.

How did you hydrate before starting this program (how much and what kinds of liquid did you drink every day)? Would you like to make changes to that pattern?

I drink some water (maybe 4 glasses/day) and know I should drink more. Sometimes I go all day without drinking anything. I like herbal and green teas and also have decaf coffee. Recently gave up alcohol, as I was drinking way too much vodka at night.

How will you hold yourself accountable for your food choices during the next six weeks?

I have been supplied with a clean-eating food list for the next six weeks by my gym. I am going to start prepping my food in bulk and keeping 3 days of meals in the refrigerator and any extra in the freezer. This way I will be able to just grab my food when it is time to eat and not have to worry about it.

I am going to keep a journal to track what I am doing and eating, as well as a 42-day countdown clock so that I can think about the weight loss challenge every day. My husband and son will also help to hold me accountable with healthy food choices.

As part of the requirement for the challenge at my gym, I had to change my Facebook status as well as to: check-in and log all workouts. At first, I was reluctant, scared, and embarrassed to do this. Like, I have to admit to the world that I am fat and want to lose weight! My friends on Facebook seem very supportive of what I am jumping into. This online workout journal that everyone can see will surely hold me accountable. It is not as scary as I thought.

WEEK 2: WHAT IS YOUR VIEW ON EXERCISE?

Have you tried (and given up on) an exercise program before starting this health-style program? What are your reasons for not starting or continuing with that past fitness program?

I have tried exercise programs many times before and never stuck with any for the long term. This includes various aerobic recordings, weight-lifting routines, walking routines, etc. I've always been strong, even though I'm heavy. When I'm not sick, I can go hiking with my husband. When my son was a baby, I would carry him in the baby backpack and hike as well. However, during the years before getting sick, I seem to have lost more and more energy (as I got heavier and heavier). It's been a real struggle.

I could never get up in the morning to exercise. Somehow my husband does though, and he also works full time. I don't know how he juggles it. Time, being tired, and maybe getting bored are the reasons I haven't stuck with it before. It wasn't until this last year with all the rehab that I've really stuck to some sort of routine to get myself out of bedrest to become stronger. I've been working hard to get my strength back and want to be stronger than I have ever been before. I've been consistently walking these past 6 months. First I was only walking in the house, then to the mailbox, then to the stop light, and after months got up to 10 miles.

What are the strengths you can use to combat any barriers to exercise?

Geez, if I knew I probably would have stuck with a program before! *Duh!*

I am now determined to make long-term changes for my own health. I can't go back to almost dying again. I would say my combined determination and persistence is a large strength to combat the part of me which sabotages my ability to stick with an exercise program.

Deep down part of me feels like a fraud trying to exercise, since I'm so big, out of shape, and physically challenged from all these damn surgeries! I can't even do half the moves everyone else can at this new gym! I'm not lean and strong like my husband and I don't have a single visible muscle and never have.

A strength that I need to tap into is the belief that I can do this and that I deserve to do this. I know somewhere inside of me that strength is there or else I would not be embarking upon this journey. Most would laugh at me if they knew that I question my own self-confidence, because they see a very different person on the outside. I just don't seem to have a lot of self-confidence for this topic. I gotta dig deep for some strength here! These new workouts are really tough!

As you start your new path, describe your health and emotional benefits from doing an exercise program.

Health benefits are huge! I am helping my joints feel better and this body will get stronger and stronger. Though right now my whole body hurts from this gym!

Exercise will help my bones (osteoporosis), and I don't want to be in my late 40s and a hunched-over old lady from full-blown menopause, as my ovaries were taken out last year. Also, a strong healthy body will help prevent cancer from coming back.

Emotional benefits: This seems to be becoming a huge inner journey, which is a little scary. I cried like a baby last week after each workout and I don't know why. I'm hoping to feel a sense of long-term inner confidence and self-esteem. Staying emotionally present is a big challenge for me as I seem to hide my inner self, and I will have to stay emotionally conscious and present in thinking about my daily health (versus putting me and my health on the back burner).

Describe your current consistency with a workout program.

I'm totally committing deeper than I have ever committed before. I'm going to the gym 5–6 times/week. I got a good jumpstart with all the rehab and home exercise this last year and now have completed a week at the gym. The routines are kicking my butt bigtime, but I haven't given up once, even though I have to modify so many exercises. And I can't do them as well as everyone else!

I want to become the person who has always been trapped inside of me. It is time to be free. It is time to live. I can stick this out for another 5 weeks and see what happens! I mean, it is only 5 more weeks! One day at a time!

Describe any social support that will hold you accountable to your new exercise program. How will *you* hold yourself accountable?

My husband and son are an amazing support crew. They want to see me happy and have helped me through everything these last few years. My hubby even has helped me shop for my food items on my current clean-eating list.

I'm committed to my Facebook check-ins for each workout. I'm also building a routine. Same hour each day for exercise, set my gym clothes out at night, eat the same meals at the same time every day. I even have my water jug ready each night for the following day.

WEEK 3: LET'S DO SOME DIGGING

Why do you continue to choose a new health-style?

I want to be fit and healthy! Working out at the gym these last two weeks has really shown me how weak I am still. I can still barely lift my legs off the ground, though I have made some progress on that front. I still feel like I'm dragging through the hour class. I want to be able to do a routine like this! Or even pull "a double" and do two classes in a row.

I don't want to put myself or my family through two years of health hell again!

What is working for you so far in this journey? What isn't working?

I've lost some weight, though not as much as I want. I worry that I won't get the 20 pounds off by the end of 6 weeks. But, the clean eating is making me feel good and the exercise is making me feel stronger.

There are some things that I could do at the end of Week 2 that I couldn't do on my first day in the gym. That is cool. Stressing about this process isn't working. I am comparing myself to others, their weight loss amount, and their progress in the gym. I have to remember that this is about me and my journey. Also, eating the same exact meal for breakfast, lunch, and dinner has not been fun. I need to have fun with this process, so I'm going to start exploring other ways to assemble and cook my meals.

How can you build on—and strengthen—what is working?

I can build on a positive and fun attitude. I have not been giving myself permission to have fun with this process and I want to loosen up a bit.

I am going to start cooking with my favorite spices, teas, etc. as I have been approaching food in a boring and bland way, and that totally isn't me! I'm going to start setting mini-goals in my workouts and focus on them, rather than mentally beating myself up for not being good enough to keep up with everyone else.

I will continue giving it my all. I also need to trust this process—and give myself credit for all the things that I am achieving in my workouts, sticking to my food plan, etc. I haven't been giving myself any credit so far. It's sad how mean I can be to myself! I'm the only one mentally beating myself up!!!

Describe your current state in terms of your feelings and attitude. Are you positive, negative, blah, energetic, tired, scared, happy, wishful, lonely, frustrated, or something else? Get it all out!

I am tired and sore. I seem to be on an emotional roller coaster these last few weeks. Happy, bitchy, tired, mad, sad, and then I cry. I feel like something inside of me is just breaking—I'm frustrated at my body.

I'm mad as hell that I got myself so unhealthy over the years. Wondering if I would have even had massive health issues if I had a healthy body to begin with? It's a "chicken and egg" situation, and I will never know which came first.

I do feel hopeful for the future and I'm trying to cling to this optimism. It can only get better and I can only get stronger. I can't quit now. There is no way I can go back to how I was!

I'm also feeling impatient. I wish this was a faster process. But then, I guess I didn't gain all this weight overnight or in a 2-week period.

How can you encourage yourself to stay on track with your new health-style?

Relax, be positive, and enjoy this journey. I need to quit focusing on the past and where I was. Rather, think about where I want to be and get there! Silence all the "should've's," "would've's," and "could've's." I can't go back in time. I can only set my path for the future.

Quit feeling like a failure with a failed and broken body, and really start working on these mini-goals—and totally celebrate and be happy about achieving them! Remember to be gentle and kind with myself like when I was in rehab. It took work to walk again, and this is gonna take work to get fit. Be nice to me!!!!

Do you believe you can achieve this and, if so, why?

Yes, I can do this. Because I am determined to see it through. I think I'm cocky for writing this down, but, by God, I f'ing deserve this. I have fought so frickin' hard to get to this point. I deserve a fit and healthy body! I'm gonna keep fighting for it.

Are there any demotivating factors or roadblocks currently in your way? If so, what can you do to remove them?

My most demotivating factor is myself—but I can't just get rid of me. I let self-doubts and insecurities get in my mind. I need to work on those, and learn to love that girl in the mirror with all the lumps and bumps and surgical scars. I need to respect my own journey. It's not about where I want to end up, it's about getting there. Life doesn't start when I get to my goal. Life is right now. I need to start really living—RIGHT NOW!

WEEK 4: EXPLORE YOUR BENEFITS

In what way do you measure the quality of your health? In what way do you measure the quality of your life? Are they the same?

I measure everything by how much physical strength and life-energy I have. For years I seemed tired ALL THE TIME, even though I worked 70-80 hours/week and juggled a husband and son. I had energy to work, but I felt like a walking zombie in other aspects of my life. I would often lie on the couch all weekend or have to pull the car over to take a nap! When lupus came out of remission and cancer hit, I spent 2 more years being tired all the time, because my body was either exhausted from being sick or exhausted from trying to recover.

I also use happiness as a measurement. I realized last year how unhappy in life, in general, I have been. I don't know who I am. I'm Mary, the cancer survivor, or childhood survivor, or Doctor Scientist, or Businesswoman, or Wife, Mom, or Daughter. But what and who am I really, besides a label? What really makes me happy and makes my heart sing with joy (besides my family)? What do I really enjoy doing? Who do I want to become? I seem to still be answering and exploring these questions.

Three weeks into this journey, I feel like I am beginning to uncover the real me that has been hiding inside of myself. I feel "present"—and this is a very new feeling.

What successes have you had on your journey thus far? What do you envision your future to look like?

I've had some great success so far. 3 weeks ago, I could not lift my legs up off the floor in front of me. (Everyone else at gym could on day 1). This week, I lifted each leg a few inches! I was in such happy tears. I showed a few new friends at the gym and they were so happy for me and gave me a huge hug! I totally felt in the moment, like I belonged at the gym, as well as feeling I had accomplished something for ME!

I'm already getting stronger with lifting the weights! I had no idea my arms were so strong. Another success is that my clothes are fitting SO MUCH looser! I've lost 12 pounds so far and feel so encouraged! My husband has given me sweet compliments (like calling me pretty) these last 15 years, but I always thought he was "just saying it." Well, this week when he called me pretty, I actually felt pretty! *Really* felt pretty. This is a first. This is a huge win! I'm even crying as I write this.

Future success will be me reaching my ultimate goal: finding the real me inside, being fit and strong, having some muscles to show for it, and being happy within. True pure happiness.

Describe any constructive or destructive behaviors which contribute to your health. Describe any outside influences (such as friends, family, work environment, etc.) which impact your overall health. How do you feel about these behaviors and influences?

In the past, when I was tired all the time, I turned to caffeine and food for energy to keep going. Too much caffeine during the day was balanced by alcohol at night to slow down, or else I couldn't sleep. I gave up caffeine and alcohol last year when the cancer surgeries started. Ending that cycle has helped, or else I might not have lost weight with all the following rehab.

However, until Three weeks ago, I still found myself turning to food when I was tired, stressed, or had something to celebrate. I have actually stuck to this new food plan so far, so no emotional eating! I've sure been tempted though! The emotional eating habits are behaviors which contribute to my health.

My attitude is a big factor too. That has actually gotten a bit better this week. I am being more positive and forgiving with myself. I started to celebrate little victories along the way and give myself credit for sticking with this for 21 days so far. (!) I'm not feeling so much like an outcast, outsider, or freak at the gym with all my physical limitations like I did a few weeks ago. In fact, I'm actually a bit proud of myself for doing this! My behaviors are in my mind.

Rehab these last few years gave me a sense of belonging, because I could *justify* being there—I had a broken body, and I had to learn how to move again. However, in "real life," I've felt sort of like a fraud when I tried a workout program (who am I, a fat chick, or an out-of-shape chick, trying to do this?). 3 weeks into this, I'm realizing that I'm DOING THE PART. I don't have to look a certain way to be on this path. Fit people don't start out fit, they work for it. My behaviors can totally change my overall health.

I'm surrounded by awesome supporting social factors. For example, my husband is a runner, eats healthy, and exercises 6 days a week. I'm a little jealous of how he can balance his life to include exercise and stay in amazing shape. I've never had the confidence to work out with him as I don't want to slow him down—or further bring to light how out of shape and weak I am.

Wow, I'm realizing that I don't even want to show those closest to me how vulnerable I can be with this topic. I seriously need some behavior adjustments! My gym environment is a great social factor contributing to my health. I am surrounded by an amazing group of people who are also on a health journey and who have all come in with their own story. I'm finding that I'm not the only one who struggles. I'm not alone! And I belong here!

What are some of the underlying needs in your life? Why are these important to you?

I don't know if this is a "need," but I am realizing: I have a hard time showing vulnerability. I don't know if this is a "trust " need, but maybe this is why I never felt like I belonged while doing fitness before, because I have to show the world that I'm not perfect. Instead, I have to admit that I have fat and weakness and am vulnerable to health and fitness topics. I'm not in control, or else I would have never gotten this way.

It seems like asking for help shows that "I can't handle it," and I feel like I'm supposed to be able to handle everything. Or maybe if I show vulnerability, I can get hurt in some way. I've been hurt so much in life. I guess this is part of trying to figure out who the real me is inside. I have a need to feel accepted. Though, over the course of these last 3 weeks, I've begun to realize that I really need to accept myself. This is where the issue lies.

I don't seem good enough for myself. Perhaps if I start accepting myself, I can really accept and believe the compliments I receive. Or accept and celebrate more accomplishments. I also have the need to "win" this. I have fought and struggled so hard to make it through so many different circumstances. Yet, I let myself down when it comes to health and wellness. If I can win this battle, perhaps I will finally be at peace with many things inside of me. Either way, I must conquer this issue.

I need to be present in life. I have spent my adult years as a zombie, just moving through the motions, going from one goal to the next, or going through one health battle to the next. I don't feel like I have slowed down to simply LIVE my life. Or to be consciously aware of who I really am. Over the years I feel like I have missed out on a lot with my husband and son, either because of career goals, or because of health battles. I'm tired of not really "living" life.

This health-style journey has forced me to think about sticking with the food and exercise plan *every* day. Also, I am thinking about a lot of topics within myself that I haven't really thought about before.

To answer the question, as I progress forward I would love to be able to look in the mirror and say "I love you" to the girl looking back at me. I have a long way to go to get here. What the hell is wrong with me? Why can't I do such a simple thing?

Describe a past situation or experience that, when you think about it, causes old feelings and behaviors to come up. How does this contribute to—or take away from—your current health-style path?

Oh hell. I'll need another journal for this one! As a child, I was "never good enough" for my mother (my parents divorced when I was 10). Nothing, I MEAN NOTHING, I did was right. If I brought home an A-, I was told that I was a stupid idiot. If I brought home an A+, I was told that I was a show off and a damned bitch. If I spent all day cleaning the kitchen and forgot to clean the crumbs from the toaster, I was beaten and called lazy.

She started putting me on diets when I was 7 years old, because she said I was fat. I even quit ballet and gymnastics, because she said I was fat and didn't look like the other girls. I didn't feel like I belonged. I never felt like I belonged *anywhere*. Except school. I escaped into academics and was good there. I thought I was a fat kid, even though when I look at pictures from childhood now, I see a perfectly normal-sized kid!

In the 9th grade the fat commentary got really bad. I was a size 9 then. In the 10th grade, I got anorexic and dropped down to a size 0, but then I was just called a slut and whore by her. I moved in with my dad in the 12th grade and graduated high school as a size 12. I shot up to a size 16 in college, then an 18/20 in graduate school.

NOTHING WAS EVER RIGHT with my mom, and I was always having to prove myself! She was a paranoid schizophrenic with multiple personality disorder, and she died from multiple sclerosis when I was 24. I don't have a single memory of her giving me a hug. All I learned from her was: "Don't be weak, or you will get attacked!" So even with lots of years of therapy and post-traumatic stress work, I guess I still have issues when it comes to the root causes of my health journey.

As a child, she would sometimes not feed me for a while as punishment, so I would hide food under my bed or in the dollhouse. Food became a reward. Like, I felt a certain power of being able to eat behind her back. When I got anorexic for that year, I felt a certain power over my body. My mom was physically abusive until around the 9th grade, which was when I could fight back. However, her boyfriend helped rob me of my childhood and was sexually abusive for many years until I moved in with my dad.

I learned through therapy years later that those who are sexually abused often find some sort of power and control through unhealthy eating habits. Shit, I'm crying as I write again.

I don't want to feel invisible anymore, like I did as a teenager. I want to feel good enough and in control of my body and mind! I want a healthy, strong body—for me! I want the power and control with my health-style. I think if I can conquer my health-style path, then I am going to conquer a lot of leftover demons from my past.

It's time that I don't hide the real me anymore, whoever/whatever that may be. I'M DONE HIDING. Fuck it, world. This mama has arrived!!!!

WEEK 5: CAN'T STOP. WON'T EVER STOP.

List every excuse and reason you can think of for NOT making your health-style a priority in your life:

Too busy in life: have to juggle work, home, parenthood, and being a wife.

Too tired and I hate getting up early: I need extra sleep.

I'm sore and it hurts.

Doubt myself and give up like I always do when it comes to this topic.

Gain a few pounds: feel like a failure, so I quit everything.

Take care of everyone else: and not care for myself.

I am all alone in this.

What actions can you take to get back on track when you start making excuses?

READ THE PREVIOUS JOURNAL ENTRIES!!! Writing here has made me realize many things about myself as well as how much support I have around me. Stay conscious of my journey. Keep tracking my workouts on the kitchen calendar and on Facebook. Tracking holds me accountable for working out.

Perhaps work out with my husband? This will help me wake up in the mornings. Having buddies in the gym also will help stay on track.

Start to fully believe in myself and continue setting mini-goals as an action plan!

Imagine getting back on track after making excuses to quit. How does this make you feel?

It feels wonderful! I feel present and in control. I feel proud for not giving up. I feel committed to my health. This is a long-term lifestyle path, not just a short-term goal with the number on the scale. I want to continue feeling great about what I'm doing for me and my health.

Who or what can stop you from achieving your goal and adopting a new health-style for the long term? What are you going to do about it?

Geez, I'm realizing that *I'm* the one who can stand in the way—me and my doubts, insecurities, lack of acceptance and love for myself. Damn, I've been working so hard though. I'm proud of me! I've come a long way and can keep on going with this path.

It sounds dumb, but I'm going to go look in the mirror and say, "I love you for sticking with it. Great job!" Hell, if I could tell my employees "great job," I should be able to tell myself the same! Or at least say, "I love the work and effort you are doing!" when I look in the mirror.

WEEK 6: MAKING IT A LIFESTYLE

What strengths have you uncovered within you?

I can apply determination, resilience, and my new confidence to this "health-style" topic. I've actually stuck with the food plan and I completed my workouts—even with high stress, I haven't quit!

I was in a car accident last week, totaled my car, and spent half the day in the emergency room, followed by 2 solid days in bed with massive soreness and a concussion. Plus, I tweaked my abdomen from the seat belt and burned my hand from the frickin' exploded air bag. (Those things hurt!)

Normally, this physical and mental stress would send me overeating. Not this time! I stuck with my plan. After 3 days rest, I went back to the gym and modified almost every exercise. Can't even lift weights, because of soreness, but I can lift my arms. So I lift my arms. I march in place. I show up. I am not going to give up after all this work! I'm not going to mindlessly shove food in my face! Not once have I felt like a failure or an outcast for having to modify EVEN MORE exercises than I normally have to.

Something inside of me has changed. I've uncovered the ability to be kind to myself at times, rather than being so demanding and hard. I'm starting to give myself recognition for my work, such as reaching mini-goals. I now feel proud to say that I've lost 50-some pounds (so far), rather than ashamed to admit it. I feel like I belong on this path *for me*.

List your top favorite "wins" since starting this new path (goals achieved, scale and/or Non-Scale Victories, etc.). Why are these significant to you?

Lifting my legs off the floor! I couldn't do this day one, but I can do it now!

Being able to jog, without stopping, to the basketball hoop and back!

Lifting 15 pounds in each hand over my head (before the car accident).

Having the energy to walk to the park with my family on the weekend!!! LOVED THIS ONE!! I ACTUALLY PLAYED AT THE PARK. My son and husband were SO HAPPY that I came along and had fun.

Really feeling pretty when my husband called me pretty.

Being able to look at myself in the mirror and even say "Good job today!"

List your top learnings/insights realized on this journey so far. Can these insights help you further? How?

It is alright—and even healing—to cry.

It's o.k. to feel vulnerable and ask for help and support. I am surrounded by love and support and need to accept it inwardly—it won't hurt me.

I have the power to change my health-style for the better.

I have the strength to achieve my fitness goals—and my goals keep getting bigger and bigger!

I have learned to accept myself and be kind to myself.

Have fun in life! And, it's o.k. to have fun in life! (Giving myself permission to have fun and be happy is huge for me.)

Surround myself with positive energy and positive people.

I feel a bit silly that it has taken me so long to realize these insights. However, I say "good for me" for realizing them. These are going to help me further, because I'm really going to start living my life this way. I have a chance for a second life after almost dying last year, and I'm taking it!

How will you continue your nutritional and exercise goals moving forward? Will you start/continue with a gym membership or exercise program? How will you integrate a healthy eating style for the long term? List your planned actions.

Keep going with the nutritional clean-eating plan. I'm not changing anything at this point, because I feel good eating this way. Plus, I want to continue to lose weight.

Integrating a healthy eating style should be easy. I just need to keep doing what I'm doing. I found that it is much easier eating clean as long as I play with spices. Cooking is fun again, because I'm exploring all the fun stuff I like to do! New recipes, new spices. I have even found many restaurants which cater to clean, healthy eating! My hubby and I have been exploring these new restaurants on date night or family outings. Also, it is fun teaching my son about healthy eating.

My exercise goals keep expanding. This week, I want to attempt double classes. That was a dream of mine during Week 1. I'm going to see if I'm strong enough to pull it off.

I want to keep increasing my strength on the weights. I would like to build some visible muscles, which seems almost laughable, since I'm so marshmallow-y. But, it is a goal and if I stick with it, I can do this!

I'm going to get a *yearly* membership at my gym. Yep, I'm committing the next 12 months to my fitness goals!

I also want to work on my walking distance outside of gym. I have always had the dream of walking 30 miles in a single day. It seems like a far-distant dream, but with a lot of work, I think I can get there some day.

Where do you want to be in your health and fitness journey, three weeks from now? Three months from now? Six months from now? One year from now?

3 weeks from now: Do double classes consistently.

3 months from now: Have the strength and endurance to lift heavier weights, lose another 15 pounds, and put some muscle on.

6 months from now: Lose inches and build muscle, join ELITE weight training class, do some sort of work out with my husband (I have always dreamed of doing P90X), walk 15 miles easily, and have my weight and BMI be in a "normal" range for the first time in my adult life.

1 year from now: DREAM LAND: Be a size 4 (last year I was a size 18/20, but I think I'll be ending next week at a size 8). Have my body fat percentage at 19-20%, which gives the toned athletic muscle-y look I dream of. (Last year I was at 54%). Be able to walk 30 miles in a day. Be super strong! Have completed the P90X program with the hubby. Start training for some athletic event.

You have one more week to go on your current six-week journey. How are you feeling? Do you have any concerns, fears, or demotivating factors? If so, list them here. Ask yourself "Why do these exist?" Now write any actions you can take to counteract them.

I'm excited and also a little scared. I have 2 pounds to go! What if I don't make it? I'm signing up for a full-year membership to my gym and need to keep my head up high and keep working toward the goals listed above. I'm doing my ultimate best, and that is all I can do!

The car accident was demotivating, but I can work around that. It won't be bothering me a few weeks from now, and I have goals to keep striving for.

I must continue being kind to myself. Also, I need to be patient with myself. It will take me time to reach my goals, so I can't mentally sabotage myself like I have done before. I can't go back into the mindset of thinking I'm a failure if I don't reach my goals overnight.

I have to remember that I am worth it! And I deserve this! And I need to keep saying all this to myself when I feel demotivated. I've come a long way!

APPENDIX C: MARY'S CONCLUSIONS (WEEK 48: MY JOURNEY IS ONLY BEGINNING)

I am writing this entry on Week 48 of my lifetime "challenge." So much has happened since my initial 6-week journey. I have now lost 75 pounds, I am within a healthy body mass index, and I am training for my first half-marathon! I continue to set mini-goals for myself and have actively participated in each of the *seven* "6-week challenges" at my gym this year.

With the first 6-week challenge (which is described in the journal entries in this book) I lost 26 pounds. I took a weeklong cruise a few days after the first challenge. I continued to workout every day and eat clean on the cruise and actually lost 3 more pounds!

When I came back from the vacation, I focused on challenge #2, where I wanted to do "double classes" (2 hours in a row) for 6 weeks. I did it! Boy, was it hard at first, but I did it!! I also had mini-goals to deadlift (a weight lifting full-body move) for 4 minutes straight and row on the rowing machine for 1 hour without stopping. Mission accomplished. I lost another 10 pounds!

Challenge #3 was a challenge within the challenge, because I had to go through another cancer surgery (a lumpectomy)—surgery #7 in all. It took a few weeks to rehabilitate after that. Luckily, it was just a lump and no cancer was detected. It was very hard emotionally to take another hit. But, I got through it and did not revert to old habits when I was stressed out. Quite the victory!

Challenge #4 was all about getting my strength and endurance back up, since it was tough to lift my arms again after surgery. I rebounded pretty fast, though. During challenge #5 I started to work on "leaning out" with the goal to lose 20 inches in 6 weeks. It was a pretty big goal. When I came to the end of the 6 weeks, I found that I had not lost a single pound—but I succeeded in losing 22 inches off my frame! This was one of my favorite challenge periods. It showed me that the scale does not rule my world! I worked up the courage to train with my husband in the mornings at this point as well. We completed 12 weeks of the Beachbody P90X program together! I did P90X in the early mornings, and went to the gym in the late morning. That began to really build my endurance, as well as my mental and physical strength. What a win, to have the confidence to workout with the hubby!

By challenge #6, I had started Elite weight training at my gym, where the workouts focused on weight lifting instead of HIIT (High Intensity Interval Training) for an hour. I also started jogging, which turned into running—which (can you believe it?) turned into training for a half-marathon. I ran 10 miles for the first time 2 weeks ago. It was a great feeling. My husband has gone on a couple runs with me, too. I'm currently in the last week of 6-week challenge #7 for the year. My goal was to run 8 miles (I beat that already!), lift heavy weight (I beat that already, too!), and drop my body fat composition to 19%. I was at 20% at the beginning of the challenge. Let's see what happens! My ultimate goal now is to get to 16% body fat composition and to feel I have a good, athletic physique.

My health-style moves forward. I am already setting goals for next year. I have registered for 3 half-marathons to keep me running for the next 9 months. Hopefully my rheumatoid arthritis and osteoarthritis will hold up. (So far, so good.) I do have some general aches and pains here and there, so I do extra rest or ice when my body tells me to. I am planning on completing the Spartan Trifecta Races toward the end of next year as well. This is my New Year's resolution coming up—as well as my 44th birthday present to myself (my birthday is in 10 months). Also, the hubby has volunteered to be my "Spartan buddy" and train with me! I'm super excited to get this going. We are already brainstorming ideas and doing research together.

I continue with physical therapy for rehabbing from all the cancer surgeries. When I started training heavy and running a few months ago, we discovered that I still have many leftover issues from all the surgeries in my core and chest. Long story short, I started overcompensating with other muscles (and pulling them). A few more months of physical therapy work and I should be good to go. Fingers crossed. I'm a work in progress. I am working hard in therapy and seeing great gains so far. I do have physical challenges still, but what would life be without challenges? I am not giving in just because I have to wrap my wrist, tape my knees, wear compression socks and sleeves, bind my core, use anti-chafing cream, or deal with colitis issues when running. No matter what, I am not going to give up! I am so grateful for my health. The cancer has not come back. The lupus remains in remission. And my joints are holding out. I am doing this! I am blessed to be alive and healthy.

I sometimes fear going back to my old habits for the long term. However, clean eating and exercise have become such a part of my life now, I simply feel "antsy" if I'm not moving and I don't feel good if I do not eat clean. There have been a few times that I have made myself sick by trying to take shortcuts (sugar alcohols in some protein bars got my inflammation going, resulting in severe gut issues) or indulging in foods which are known to cause me inflammation (cane sugar and soy are found in most chocolates). I know I still have "hummingbird cravings" with sugar. What a power sugar has over me. I know it causes inflammation in my body, but I still crave it. I have to consciously say "NO" and walk away. The struggle is real. I think this will always hang in the background and tempt me. I have to stay mentally prepared for it! Yes, yes, yes, there are times that I go off-plan. Yes, I have cheat meals here and there. That is life. *This* is life. You gotta live your life. But, I can live my life in a healthy manner now. I am taking care of me. This is the first time that I have *really* taken care of me, physically, mentally, and spiritually for over a year!

I continue many different tricks to hold myself accountable. I monitor my weight on the scale on a weekly basis. I still track my gym workouts and "check in" on Facebook. Today was the 172nd time that I have gone to the gym since starting my first 6-week challenge! (I only count 1 check-in per day at the gym, because it would get too crazy if I counted every double class or extra things that I do!) I had set the goal to check in 200 times at the end of the first challenge described in this journal. I also write my running mileage on the calendar for every run that I do. I set very specific SMART goals for each 6-week challenge at my gym.

I am now setting specific long-term goals (such as the half-marathons and Spartan races) to keep carrying my training forward. One of my primary reasons to train for this upcoming January half-marathon (it is December at the time of this journal entry) is to keep me moving during the holiday season! I did not want to start making excuses and fall off my training plan over the holidays, and end up gaining a bunch of weight back. I even enlisted a few gym friends to join me on this half-marathon running adventure. I really can't quit now, because my friends are training too! I have found that, for me, self-accountability and sharing accountability with friends is a key component to maintaining this lifestyle. My suggestion for you is to surround yourself with like-minded people—and a positive environment!

I have learned so much in this last year. Many of the thoughts, feelings, and lessons learned in the 42 days of my first 6-week journey are the very nuggets that have carried me forward to now. I have learned to believe in my health-style path, and to believe that I truly deserve a healthy and happy life. I have learned that I am not alone in this process, and that this is a lifetime process!

I had to dig really deep within and think about issues from my past that I do not usually think about. However, as I move through my new lifestyle, I found much-needed peace with many aspects of my past. With this peace, I am finding that I am less apt to fall into old self-defeating habits around nutrition and fitness. Now, I am not perfect at all. Just this last weekend, I began beating myself up because I "only" ran 7 miles and my goal was 11 miles. I dropped into my old perfectionist self, the old "I'm not good enough unless I overachieve all the time" self, the old "you are such a loser because you didn't make it" self. I was really starting to beat myself up over this "failed" run. My lovely husband brought me back to reality, by pointing out how awesome 7 miles is, how far I have come, etc. It didn't take me long at all to realize that I was using this one run to begin to sink back into old habits. I was able to shake out of it and be kind to myself, and actually celebrate that I am out on the road, running. I celebrated my victory with an awesome haircut that made me feel sexy—I didn't have to eat a bunch of gluten-free brownies to celebrate! The old me would have never even recognized the self-bashing behavior! The old me also would have never listened and internally accepted the praise from my husband, because I did not think I was good enough. The old me would have over-indulged in the gluten-free brownies as comfort as I was feeling bad for bashing myself. I am good enough now. I know it. I embrace it. I love the woman that I have found within me. No more hiding. *Never again.* I don't need to hide under a big girl. I love me. This woman is here. I am finally beginning to get to know myself. I deserve to be healthy and fit!

The work I did to learn to be able to trust and to feel and show vulnerability still carry me through today as well. I actually feel closer to my husband, as well as to my friends around me, because I am more open, more accepting of myself, and more at peace. I am simply being and living as "me" instead of trying to be the "what is expected" version of me. This openness has also put me in a nice space to be able to mentor others. In fact, my business school recently asked me to be an executive mentor to some students. I am very excited to be able to give back and help others. My gym also recently asked me to be an ambassador for our location—another opportunity to give back to others. The benefits of this health-style journey are actively pouring over into other areas of my life in a very good way.

My journey is only beginning. I can't wait to see where I am this time next year!!

ABOUT THE AUTHOR

Mary A. Tichi, Ph.D., MBA is the founder and current owner of Micronostics, a consulting company focused on helping people to create their own strategic paths to health, wellness, and overall personal and professional well-being.

In her role as fitness mentor and ambassador for her local gym, Mary brings 22+ years of experience including teaching, coaching, and mentoring in strategic operations, business and commercial development, and sales and marketing.

Mary has taken a difficult set of circumstances and not only has made a positive change in herself, but she continues to inspire that same shift in thinking (and living!) in others. Her own trials and triumphs speak to those who have also been struggling and her experience gives a unique and valuable perspective that is easy to trust. Mary has an openness that shines through her advice, nudging others to have confidence in what is best for them and their own bodies.

Mary's authorship was inspired after her two-year battle with lupus and breast cancer, a time that led her to clean eating, exercise, and acknowledgment of her own inner strength. Upon losing 75 pounds and winning her health battles, she has learned the importance of channeling her energy on living a good, positive life, with the same focus it took to receive a BS in (Medical) Microbiology at the University of Washington, a doctorate in Microbiology (Plant Biotechnology) from The Ohio State University, and a Master's of Business Administration from the Rady School of Management,University of California-San Diego.

Mary was born and raised in the great Pacific Northwest, in the Seattle, Washington, area. Since 2004, Mary has resided in the San Diego, California, area. She currently lives in Carlsbad (CA), with her husband, son, and two beloved cats.